PLANT, ABIOTIC STRESS AND RESPONSES TO CLIMATE CHANGE

Edited by **Violeta Andjelkovic**

Plant, Abiotic Stress and Responses to Climate Change
http://dx.doi.org/10.5772/intechopen.69916
Edited by Violeta Andjelkovic

Contributors

Marina Putnik-Delic, Ivana Maksimovic, Nevena Nagl, Branislava Lalić, Carla António, Tiago F. Jorge, Luis Rubén García-Dávila, Adalberto Benavides Mendoza, Hipólito Hernández-Hernández, Fabián Pérez-Labrada, Ema Laura García Enciso, Paola Leija-Martínez, Mari Carmen López-Pérez, Julia Medrano-Macías, Susana González-Morales, Antonio Juarez Maldonado, Luis Rodriguez-Zapata, Evelyn Arlette Carrillo-Bermejo, Samuel Gamboa-Tuz, Miguel Ángel Herrera-Alamillo, Manuel L. Robert, Enrique CastaÃ±o, Miguel A. Keb-Llanes, Zhao, Muqadas Aleem, Ripa Akter Sharmin, Phetole Mangena, Yasuo Yamauchi, Violeta Andjelkovic

First published in London, United Kingdom, 2018 by IntechOpen
IntechOpen is the global imprint of INTECHOPEN LIMITED, registered in England and Wales, registration number: 11086078, The Shard, 25th floor, 32 London Bridge Street
London, SE19SG – United Kingdom
Printed in Croatia

British Library Cataloguing-in-Publication Data
A catalogue record for this book is available from the British Library

Additional hard copies can be obtained from orders@intechopen.com

Plant, Abiotic Stress and Responses to Climate Change, Edited by Violeta Andjelkovic
p. cm.
Print ISBN 978-1-78923-122-9
Online ISBN 978-1-78923-123-6

For EU product safety concerns:
IN TECH d.o.o., Prolaz Marije Krucifikse Kozulić 3, 51000 Rijeka, Croatia,
info@intechopen.com or visit our website at intechopen.com.

Meet the editor

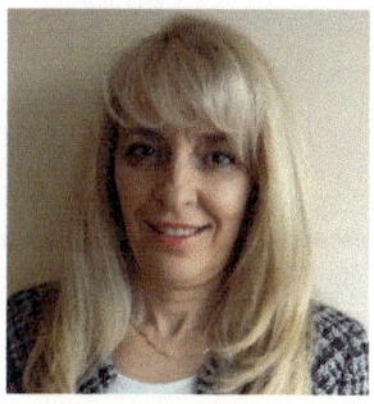

Violeta Andjelkovic obtained her PhD degree in Agronomy in the fields of genetics and plant breeding. She is the head of maize gene bank and a manager of the European maize database at the Maize Research Institute, Zemun Polje, Serbia. As a postdoctoral researcher at the Max Planck Institute, Cologne, Germany, she worked on the expression analysis of genes induced by abiotic stresses in maize. She has coauthored more than 200 publications and participated in numerous national and bilateral projects. Her actual research interest focuses on physiological and molecular aspects of abiotic stress, particularly drought, and on the improvement of drought tolerance and grain quality in maize by the utilization of genetic resources.

Contents

Preface

Climate change models predicted that crop production will decline in most production areas and will seriously affect food security in the coming decades. The world population is expected to exceed 10 billion by 2100. During the last century, agriculture fulfilled the growing demand for food by increasing the crop yield. Projections are that global warming will make changes in precipitation, together with more frequent droughts and floods; runoff in snowmelt; increase in CO_2, temperature, and evapotranspiration; reduction in water availability; and leaching of soil nutrients. Under changed climate, further increase in crop yield will not be sufficient in a growing food demand.

Although it is difficult to have accurate data of the impact of abiotic stress on crop yields, the influence is significant, according to the affected area (FAO estimations are that only 3.5% of the global arable area is not affected by some abiotic stress factors). Among all abiotic stresses, drought is going to have the most important influence on the decrease of crop production. Yield of the three most important food crops (wheat, rice, and maize) is expected to decrease in most arable areas, based on reductions in available water and increased temperature. The main tasks for researchers are to increase food production by developing sustainable agricultural practices, increase abiotic and biotic stress tolerance in crops, and introduce new crops adapted for changed conditions and environments.

The present book is comprised of two parts: the first one focuses on tolerance and adaptation of some crops (soybean, sugar beet, and sugarcane) to water stress, and the second one explains the possibilities and techniques that could help crops in reducing damages caused by global climate changes.

Soybean is the most important legume and is at the fourth place according to global crop production areas. The importance of this crop in response to climate changes lies in its biological fixation of nitrogen too. Chapter 2 presented the anatomical and morphological changes in different soybean cultivars in response to different levels of water stress. Chapter 3 pointed out the possibilities in nature among the genetic diversity and wild relatives of soybean, which could be used to alleviate global warming. Sugar beet and sugarcane are important for sugar production in different regions of the world based on climatic conditions. Sugar beet is produced more in Europe and needs an adequate amount of water for achieving a satisfactory yield. In Chapter 4, different sugar beet genotypes are tested for water stress tolerance under greenhouse conditions. Although sugarcane is C_4 crop growing in tropical regions, its production is also dependent on water availability. In Chapter 5, some new biotechnology approaches are explained in order to mitigate the effect of water stress on sugarcane production.

Besides the efforts on understanding the mechanisms of plant responses to abiotic stresses and breeding crops with increased tolerance and adaptation to climate changes, which is presented in Chapter 6 of this book, it is necessary to look for some sustainable methods and agricultural practice to obtain stable crop yields in the coming decades. The advantages of application of chemicals and biostimulants, together with traditional agricultural practice in alleviation of climate change effects on crop production, are presented in Chapter 7. Since different abiotic stresses are affecting plant growth simultaneously, plant response is very complex and difficult to predict and breed for improved tolerance to abiotic stresses. Finally, Chapter 8 gives an overview of the different stressors and mechanisms of crop response to them, with recommended agricultural techniques that could be used to help plants to survive and bring yield in spite of the negative effects of the upcoming climate change.

We are grateful to all the authors for their contributions. We express our special thanks and appreciation to Ms. Kristina Kardum, Publishing Process Manager, for her encouragement and help in bringing out the book in the present form.

Dr. Violeta Andjelkovic
Maize Research Institute
Zemun Polje, Serbia

Section 1

Introduction

Chapter 1

Introductory Chapter: Climate Changes and Abiotic Stress in Plants

Violeta Andjelkovic

Additional information is available at the end of the chapter

http://dx.doi.org/10.5772/intechopen.76102

1. Climate change

Climate change is a problem with the highest priority facing the mankind today, influencing agricultural production worldwide. According to IPCC [1], human activities are the main factor for changes that are unique over decades to millennia. Gas emissions have increased since 1950s, reach the highest level nowadays than ever. Atmospheric concentration of CO_2 was less than 300 ppm from the beginning of human civilization to 1900. The present level at about 400 ppm was not reached in more than 400,000 years. The period from 1983 to 2012 was the warmest 30-year period of the last 1400 years in the Northern Hemisphere. The Earth's average temperature increased for 1.4°C in twentieth century and is predicted to increase about 11.5°C in twenty-first century. With more climate disruption by human activities, average temperature is predicted to rise in twenty-first century, heat waves are going to be more frequent and last longer, as well as occurrence of unevenly distributed precipitation in many areas. Warming and acidification of oceans will continue, followed by rising sea levels due to the melting of polar ice, and additional rainfall leads to flooding. Climate change caused by humans is significantly faster than natural global climate change during the past millions of years and most plants cannot naturally adapt according to fast changes of ecosystems caused by global warming. Temperature increases of about 4°C in late twentieth century, is reducing wheat, rice, and maize global production and with increasing food demand, seriously affecting food security. The consequences of global warming on crop production became a major task for researchers in the past decades. Also, climate change affects a number of days when plants can grow, by their decreasing of 11% until 2100. Simultaneously, extreme temperatures and rainfalls, lowering of available water, and changes in soil quality are expected to make difficulties for plants to grow and survive. Nevertheless, plants will be exposed to different abiotic and biotic stresses at the same time and their responses will be more complex with overlapping of different stress response pathways.

2. Abiotic stress

Abiotic stress is defined as environmental factors that affect plants and reduce growth and yield below optimum levels. Plant abiotic stress factors include extremes in temperature, water, nutrients, gasses, wind, radiation, and other environmental conditions. Plant responses to abiotic stresses are dynamic and complex; they are both elastic (reversible) and plastic (irreversible). Since the plants are exposed to a combination of different stresses, responses are more complex and different stress pathways overlap [2]. In "Adapting Crops to Climate Change," the authors suggest "the major abiotic stresses expected to increase in response to climate change are drought, heat, salinity, and inundation" [3]. Nowadays, tolerance to drought and heat, and water use efficiency are receiving the most attention in breeding programs worldwide.

2.1. Drought

Drought is expected to have the highest influence on crop productivity decrease in the frame of upcoming global warming. Predictions are that 30% of land will be exposed to extreme drought by the end of twentieth century [4]. Consequently, demand for irrigation will considerably increase in future, since about 70% of water worldwide is used in agriculture. Limited resources of irrigation water will require careful management to obtain crop production for food and feed. Various plant drought responses are classified into three categories, more than 50 years ago: drought escape, drought avoidance, and drought tolerance [5].

Plants escape drought by fast phenological development, completing their life cycle before the water deficit occurs and it is distinct from drought resistance. Drought avoidance is based on plant maintenance of water status through improvement of water balance by increased water uptake by deeper roots and/or reducing water loss by increasing leaf waxiness. Drought tolerance involves biochemical mechanisms activated after stress to enable plant to maintain functional growth under low available water. Osmotic adjustment is a typical physiological mechanism for dehydration tolerance or turgor maintenance by accumulation of osmoprotectants, ABA or increase of antioxidative and other protecting mechanism. Usually, plants combined different drought responses, and their adaptation and productivity depend on balance between all three strategies. Drought tolerance is a quantitative, complex trait, under genetic control and significant influence of the environment. Despite the increasing knowledge on plant stress responses and the advancement of "omics" technologies to screen number of genes involved in drought response, the improvement in breeding for drought tolerant crops is relatively modest.

3. A system biology perspective

Recent achievements in biotechnology have significantly increased possibilities for gene discovery and functional genomics. Comprehension of gene action is a major challenge in postgenomic era, since many of the roles of particular genes are unknown, they are inferred and associated with other known genes, and that provide a better understanding of biological functioning. High throughput "omics" technologies are enabling the identification of new genes and their function. Three systematic approaches or "omics" improved our knowledge of the complex mechanisms that regulate genes and networks in stress response through adaptation and/or tolerance. The first "transcriptomics" includes the analysis of coding and noncoding RNAs, and their expression profiles. The second one "metabolomics" analyzes a large number of metabolites. The third one is "proteomics" in which protein and protein profiles offer a widening of knowledge about regulatory networks. The combination of data on gene expression, protein synthesis, and production of small cell metabolites give better overview of plant response to drought-stressed environment. System biology examines all factors in plants in response to environmental stresses that help in better explanation and understanding of involved mechanism. Integration of "omics" technologies allows identification of molecular study of abiotic stress signaling and application of biotechnology in crop production in future [6, 7].

4. Perspectives

As climate change includes crop adaptation to new environmental conditions, breeders are challenged to breed for new unpredictable conditions, and to consider the genetic potential of past breeding work. "Traits that may not have been as attractive 10, 15 or 20 years ago are more important today because with these new techniques and abilities breeders are able to look at what's in their library and although they maybe couldn't tease out a specific trait previously, today they are able to" [3]. Global warming indicates necessity to look for crops that are more convenient for new environment, not only to focus on adapted crops and attempt to improve their tolerance to drought, cold, heat, or any other emerged conditions. "If you want to talk about real sustainability it is not just about making crops that are currently the emphasis…better, it's also thinking about the big picture and what other crops we are going to need to make better to fit into those cropping systems" [3]. Progress in breeding for improved drought tolerance will be accomplished by integration of conventional breeding with physiology and genomics [8]. Large amount of available data obtained from "omics" technologies put a new challenge for agricultural bioscience in their analysis and practical applications. Developing tools integrating environmental stressors and diverse genetic backgrounds, together with numerous levels of analysis will help in better understanding of biological processes in plants under stress. Although new technics can be used to predict some aspect of plant responses to stress, there is still a large gap between huge amount of available data and our understanding of biological networks and phenomena. It required having close collaboration of agronomists, molecular biologists, biochemists, and computer scientists in order to provide those answers [9].

Author details

Violeta Andjelkovic

Address all correspondence to: avioleta@mrizp.rs

Maize Research Institute Zemun Polje, Belgrade, Serbia

References

[1] IPCC. Climate Change 2014: Synthesis Report. 2014. Available from: http://www.ipcc.ch/report/ar5/syr/ [Accessed: February 25, 2018]

[2] Fujita M, Fujita Y, Noutoshi Y, Takahashi F, Narusaka Y, Yamaguchi-Shinozaki K, Shinozaki K. Crosstalk between abiotic and biotic stress responses: A current view from the points of convergence in the stress signaling networks. Current Opinion in Plant Biology. 2006;**9**:436-442. DOI: 10.1016/j.pbi.2006.05.014

[3] Breeding for Climate Change. Available from: http://sbc.ucdavis.edu/files/206899.pdf [Accessed: February 25, 2018]

[4] Burke EJ, Brown SJ, Christidis N. Modeling the recent evolution of global drought and projections for the twenty-first century with the Hadley Centre climate model. Journal of Hydrometeorology. 2006;**7**:1113-1125. DOI: 10.1175/JHM544.1

[5] Levitt J. Responses of Plants to Environmental Stresses. New York: Academic Press; 1972. 698 p. DOI: 10.1126/science.177.4051.786

[6] Cramer GR, Urano K, Delrot S, Pezzotti M, Shinozaki K. Effect of abiotic stress on plants: A systems biology perspective. BMC Plant Biology. 2011;**11**:163. DOI: 10.1186/1471-2229-11-163

[7] Shanker AK, Maheswari M, Yadav SK, Desai S, Bhanu D, Attal NB, Venkateswarlu N. Drought stress responses in crops. Functional & Integrative Genomics. 2014;**14**(1):11-22. DOI: 10.1007/s10142-013-0356-x

[8] Stikić R, Jovanović Z, Prokić L. Mitigation of plant drought stress in a changing climate. Botanica Serbica. 2014;**38**(1):35-42. UDK 581.6:632.112

[9] Humbert S, Subedi S, Cohn J, Zeng B, Bi YM, Chen X, Zhu T, McNicholas PD, Rothstein S. Genome-wide expression profiling of maize in response to individual and combined water and nitrogen stresses. BMC Genomics. 2013;**14**:3. DOI: 10.1186/1471-2164-14-3

Section 2

Plant Tolerance to Abiotic Stress

Water Stress: Morphological and Anatomical Changes in Soybean (*Glycine max* L.) Plants

Phetole Mangena

Additional information is available at the end of the chapter

http://dx.doi.org/10.5772/intechopen.72899

Abstract

Water stress is one of the most important physiological stress factors that adversely affect soybeans in many critical aspects of their growth and metabolism. Soybean's growth, development and productivity are severely diminished, when soil or cell water potential becomes inadequate to sustain metabolic functioning. However, little has been done to gather comprehensive information regarding the specific changes that occur in water-stressed plants at the anatomical and morphological level. In this study, deviations in root growth, shoot growth, stomatal conductance, yield components and anatomical features are reported. Treatments with two levels of water stress imposed by reducing irrigation (once in 7 days or once in 15 days) revealed that, all cultivars (Dundee, LS 677, LS 678, TGx 1740-2F, TGx 1835-10E and Peking) were highly susceptible to prolonged water stress, exhibiting severe dehydration and death. A 15.0 and 30.0% survival frequency was obtained in plants irrigated once in 7 days; LS 677 and Peking, respectively. Unlike many other stresses, water deficit did not only affect the density of stomata, but, photosynthesis was affected by the lower levels of tissue CO_2. These results suggest that, balanced biochemical, physiological, anatomical and morphological regulations are necessary for increased growth and yields in soybean.

Keywords: anatomy, growth, morphology, soybean, water stress

1. Introduction

Water stress is one of the most important constraints in the growth and development of plants. Water deficit stress, in particular, is a major problem in agriculture and most crop plants show high sensitivity to this kind of stress than any kind of abiotic constraint conditions. Crop plant growth and yields are severely impacted by inadequate supply of water, which result in decreased carbon assimilates contents. In addition, plants exposed to prolonged shortage in ground, surface or atmospheric water, known as drought are highly susceptible to pests and diseases. Mattson and Haack [1] provided evidence on the occurrence of fungi and insect induced stalk rots, wilts and foliar diseases in plants caused by drought stress. The prevalence in disease outbreak occurred in water-stressed plants compared to the normal water stress-free plants. Estimations of yield losses in soybeans compiled by Wrather and Koenning in the United States from 1996 until 2007 indicated that, the role of pathogens such as soybean cyst nematode, phytophthora root and stem rot, as well as charcoal rot that affected seedling development was exacerbated by the physical environmental stress conditions [2]. Drought is, and continues to be an insidious hazard to plants, animals and human lives. Drought conditions in many regions worldwide are worsening due to various factors, some of which are caused by climate change. The increase in atmospheric CO_2 level, currently estimated at about 380–400 ppm, and alterations in hydrological cycles make drought a recurring natural hazard world-wide [3, 4]. In this regard, plants undergo permanent or temporary damage to their morphological architecture, and their anatomical and physiological processes when exposed to dry and hot conditions. According to Shao et al. [5], water stress effects can be extended in plants to alter gene expression, change cellular metabolism, cause reduction in mitotic cell division activities in mesophyll tissues and other organs, as well as to cause the decrease in stomatal conductance [6]. Scientific research showed that; drought stress causes imbalances in the natural status of the environment and drastically disrupts crop cultivation thus, threatening food security [7, 8]. Many regions have experienced the detrimental and severe effects of drought, particularly, populations in the developing countries. In the Southern African Development Community (SADC) region; poor rainfall conditions were recorded for the 2016/2017 agricultural season as a result of El Niño induced drought [9]. FAO's global information and early warning system in 2015 reported significant drought dating back to 1984 [10]. The area data covered regions such as the United States, Semi-Arido of Brazil, Eastern Europe and African countries where, severe drought causing food crisis across Ethiopia, Kenya and Somalia resulted into the deaths of over 1 million people. Therefore, the continuing drop into below-normal annual rainfalls and increasing temperatures create the relevance to study and understand the morphological/anatomical changes that plants undergo to cope with environmental stresses. In cultivated crops such as soybean (*Glycine max* L.), this would minimise limitations that adversely affect plant growth, and the improvement of this crop for yield purposes [11], as well as counteracting against factors that negatively influence the nutritional content and essential secondary metabolites synthesised in this plant.

2. Analyses of soybean responses to water deficit stress

Plants experience water deficit stress when the amount of water in the cells and surrounding becomes limiting to growth and development. To investigate these effects, a study was conducted to primarily assess the influence of water stress on the growth of soybean; morphologically and anatomically, under greenhouse conditions. According to Lisar et al. [8] water deficit is caused by prolonged water shortage. In order to examine this stress, reduction in the frequency of irrigation was performed by limiting watering to once a week (WT 1) and once in 15 days (WT 2). Plants used for the control were watered daily, depending on soil moisture content in the plastic pots. For the growth of soybean plants, plastic containers filled with a mixture of 4:1 (v/v) fertile sandy-loam soil with vermiculite was used. Seeds of soybean cultivar Dundee, LS 678, LS 677, TGx 1740-2F, TGx 1835-10E and Peking were inoculated into the pots for germination and seedling emergence. At least one soybean plant was grown per pot with 20 replicates per cultivar, and allowed to grow up to V3 stage before imposing water stress. The morphological and physiological data were then recorded, which included plant height, number of leaves plant-1, number of braches plant-1, yield and yield components, average leaf area, root length and the micro-morphological characteristics of the stomata and trichomes were evaluated. Assessment of these characteristics was guided by the methods according to Cornelissen et al. [12] with modifications. To study stomatal and trichomes characteristics the microscopic slides were prepared by a protocol modified from Yeung's [13] guide to study plant structures. Leaves of soybean plants from both the control and water-stressed plants (WT 1 and WT 2) were collected a week before the experiment was terminated. The experiment was terminated when the plants reached reproductive stage 4 (R4) of fruiting, involving maturity and seed filling. The free hand sectioning method by Yeung was used to study structural organisation of the root and stems, with section staining done using Toluidine blue O stain. Quantifying the chlorophyll content and leaf area is an important measurement for comparing plant growth, treated with different growth conditions. For leaf area assessment, leaf samples were randomly detached from the different cultivars, and their leaf area estimated as described by Richter et al. [14]. Leaves were randomly sampled for estimation of chlorophyll content using a CCM 200 plus Chlorophyll Meter, Opti-Sciences.

3. Description of soybean morphology and anatomy

Plants are responsible for a number of essential ecological services. Plants are the main primary source of foods for humans and animals, supply oxygen, timber, medicine and also have ornamental value. The multiple and complex processes involving genetic, morphological, anatomical, physiological and biochemical mechanisms are responsible for the goods and services that plants provide. These functions are made possible by the architecture of the plant's internal and external structures. Soybeans like other legumes and non-leguminous plants display different types of internal and external growth forms that functions together to provide these services. The external form include indeterminate, determinate and semi-determinate morphological growth habits, which typically take place in both the early and late maturity groups of varieties grown for commercial and subsistence farming [15]. Soybean plants with determinate growth terminate their vegetative growth stage during the onset of the reproductive stage. In contrast, indeterminate varieties continue growing even during flower setting and anthesis. Anthesis is the period in which flowers developed during the reproductive stage of the plant's life cycle begin to open. According to the NDSU [15] the semi-determinate growth habit lies between the polarity and growth of the other two growth habits (determinate and indeterminate form). The vegetative parts of soybean include the stem, leaves and the soil submerged roots. A few types of leaves can be found in soybean.

The plant has trifoliate leaves, which are photosynthetic foliage with three leaflets. They have protective scale leaves which covers and protect young immature flowers before anthesis.

These scales are small bracts which appear subtending the yellow or purple flowers of soybeans [16]. The special leaf types constituting the floral parts or inflorescence (raceme) can also be found. The vegetative stage is furthermore characterised by erect elongated stems, axillary buds, some viewed immediately above the cotyledons at the axil, unifoliate buds and the terminal buds (**Figure 1a–c**). Both young and old stems of soybeans are heavily covered by the epidermal hairs (trichomes) (**Figure 1d**). Even though soybean plants produce primary roots, originating from the seedling's embryo; the roots have many branching secondary roots that slightly resemble fibrous root system in monocots. Most of the lateral roots are concentrated at the upper part of the root zone. As in most of the dicotyledonous plants, soybean's body is made up of the three main tissue systems: dermal, ground and vascular (**Figure 1e**, **f**). The epidermis as the dermal tissue is the

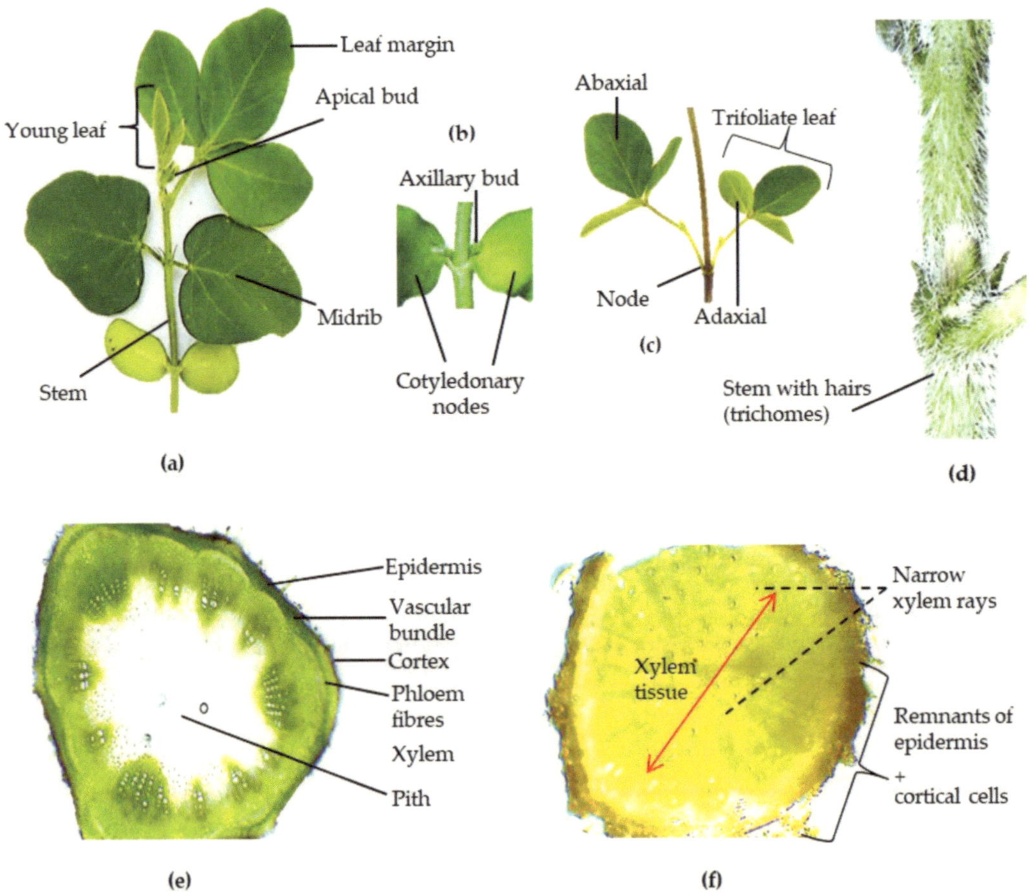

Figure 1. Overview of soybean plant morphology and anatomy. (a) Vegetative first trifoliate (V1) stage. (b) Example of cotyledons and axillary buds at the axil. (c) Trifoliate leaves showing adaxial-abaxial leaf surfaces. (d) Example of soybean stem with epidermal hairs. (e) A micrograph of soybean stem cross-section. (f) A micrograph of soybean root cross-section.

outermost single layer of cells derived from the protoderm, and in soybean it covers the plant for its entire life cycle. The three main types of epidermal cells found in soybean include trichomes and microscopic guard cells as well as the subsidiary cells of the stomata (**Figure 2b–d**). This layer of elongated and compactly arranged cells functions to protect soybean against water loss and harsh external environmental factors, including pathogens. Trichomes are unicellular or multicellular hairs occurring on shoot system of plants. On the roots, hairs are called root hairs. In leaves, this layer of cells is followed by the palisade parenchyma and spongy mesophylls.

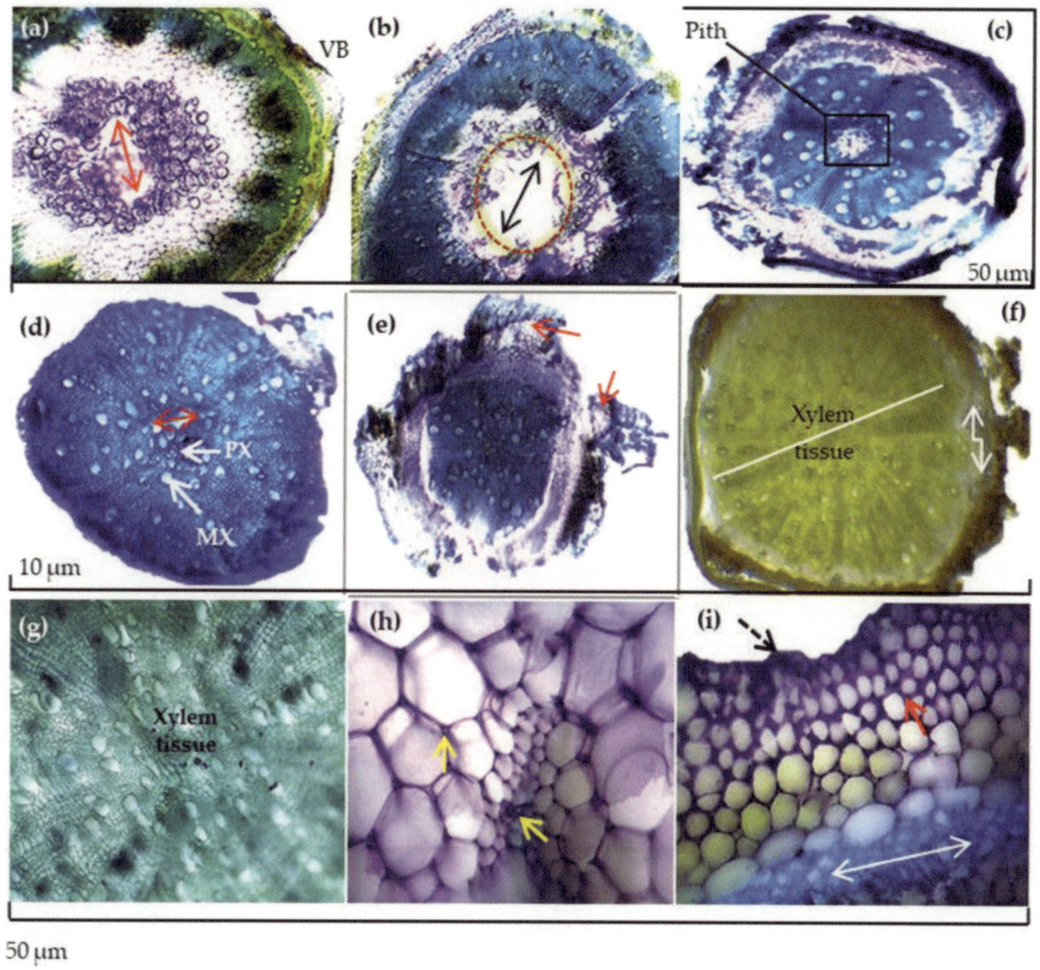

Figure 2. Examples of microscopic cross-section in roots and stems of soybean plants. (a) Formation of pith canal as a result of water stress in WT 1 plants. (b) Broadening of canal and changes on stem cortex tissue in WT 2. (c) Control plants showing unaffected pith and cortex. (d) Cross-section of WT 2 root showing rupturing of the stele, protoxylem (PX) and metaxylem (MX). (e) Cross-section of WT 1 root showing marks of lateral roots (left right arrow). (f) Root section taken from the control showing expanded thickened xylem tissue and reduced cortex. (g) Close view of xylem tissue from the control plant. (h) Close view of parenchymatous pith as indicated on (c), (arrows indicate intercellular spaces of the parenchyma. (i) Soybean cortical tissue of the stem showing phloem fibres (left right arrow), collenchyma (solid arrow) and a single layer of epidermis (dashed arrow).

The palisade and spongy cells are specialised tissues used by all eudicot plants with C_3 pathway for photosynthesis and gaseous exchange in leaves, respectively [17]. Soybean is one of the C_3 plants which undergo photosynthetic carbon reduction and do not have a CO_2 concentrating mechanism. It differs with grain crops such as maize, rice, sorghum and wheat C_4 plants that concentrate CO_2 by not salvaging carbon lost during photorespiratory carbon oxidation (PCO) cycle [17]. But, the palisade and spongy tissues of soybean form the mesophyll, a ground tissue system of a leaf, which plays a critical role in carboxylation, reduction and regeneration processes during photosynthesis. In roots and stems, the fundamental (ground) tissue consists of non-protective and non-conductive simple cells of parenchyma, collenchyma and sclerenchyma (**Figure 2e** and **f**). Evert and Eichhorn [18] referred to this tissue system as the one most dominated by parenchyma cells, which are by far considered the most common ground tissue of the pith and cortex in roots and stems of soybean and other eudicots, as well as in the monocots. The vascular system is made up of conducting strands of phloem and xylem. These are principal water and food conducting tissue in all vascular seedless and seed plants.

3.1. Morphological changes due to water deficit stress

The morphological evidence gathered in this study has shown that soybean growth is highly sensitive to water deficit stress. All plants exposed to water deficit presented significant changes in their shoot and root morphology. Complete reduction in the number of new branches per plant, initiation of leaves and expansion of the lamina (measured by estimated leaf area) and the number of trifoliate leaves per plant was observed. Decreases in the assessed morphological characteristics were more predominant in plants subjected to stress for longer periods (WT 2) than those watered once a week (WT 1). Soybean cultivar Dundee, TGx 1740-2F, TGx 1835-10E and Peking produced significantly similar mean number of trifoliate leaves (about 4.0–5.0) in WT 2, when compared to about 5.0–6.0 trifoliate leaves obtained in WT 1 (**Table 1**). Leaf rolling and flipping were observed in some of the older leaves as a result of induced water stress. The negative effects of water stress on new leaf and branch formation was also reported by Mabulwana [16]. Jaleel et al. [19] similarly added that, water stress decreases the elongation and expansion of stems and leaves. In contrast to observations made in all water stressed plants, the control exhibited normal shoot growth and the highest number of trifoliate leaves (**Table 1**).

According to Nosalewicz and Lipiec [20] suppression on the growth and distribution of the roots by water stress could also lead to the reduction in shoot growth. As the vegetative shoot growths appeared diminished by induced stress, roots in water-stressed plants became more elongated and branched than in the control. Root phenotype in the control appeared shallow and less branched than in WT 1 and WT 2 plants. However, plants which had irrigation reduced to once in 15 days (WT 2) had deep root phenotype compared to plants irrigated once a week (WT 1). Insufficient water supply for WT 2 plants with deep root development, and moderately stressed plants (WT 1), both demonstrated clear morphological changes. All cultivars in WT 2 also exhibited severe nutrient deficiency symptoms (the entire leaf with chlorosis and marginal necrosis) and stem wilting. These symptoms were accompanied by adverse growth effects and survival frequency of 0% when the experiment was terminated (**Table 2**). Water deficit stress ultimately led to the severe damage to shoots of WT 2 plants, with no possible indication of recovery. In WT 1 plants, moderate to severe deficiency symptoms

Soybean genotypes	Treatment plants 1			Treatment plants 2			Control plants		
	Mean no. of fully developed trifoliate leaves	Average leaf area (cm^2)	Stomatal density (no. of stomata/ cm^2)	Mean no. of fully developed trifoliate leaves	Average leaf area (cm^2)	Stomatal density (no. of stomata/cm^2)	Mean no. of fully developed trifoliate leaves	Average leaf area (cm^2)	Stomatal density (no. of stomata/ cm^2)
Dundee	5.0^{a}	55.1^{a}	213^{a}	5.0^{a}	55.1^{a}	112^{a}	13.0^{a}	50.0^{a}	247^{a}
LS 677	7.0^{b}	38.6^{b}	191^{b}	6.5^{b}	32.1^{b}	106^{b}	14.5^{b}	41.1^{b}	213^{b}
LS 678	6.0^{c}	40.1^{c}	203^{c}	6.0^{c}	32.1^{b}	167^{c}	13.5^{c}	57.7^{c}	212^{c}
Peking	8.0^{d}	43.9^{d}	181^{d}	4.5^{d}	36.5^{c}	143^{d}	15.5^{d}	33.6^{d}	256^{d}
TGx 1740-2F	6.0^{c}	37.5^{e}	154^{e}	5.0^{a}	40.1^{d}	163^{e}	12.5^{e}	16.1^{e}	163^{e}
TGx 1835-10E	6.0^{c}	60.1^{f}	167^{f}	4.0^{e}	30.7^{e}	155^{f}	11.0^{f}	39.8^{f}	171^{f}

The leaf area of central individual leaflets in soybean cultivars were estimated using the general Eq. LA = k × (L.W) where LA, leaf area; k, is the 'adjustment factor' estimated by linear regression forcing the regression intercepting line to be zero using Table Curve software (Richter et al. [14]), L, length of the leaflet and W, leaflet width.

Values within columns followed by different alphabets are statistically significant at $p \leq 0.05$ confidence level. For Water Treatment 1 (WT 1), irrigation frequency was reduced to once a week (After 7 days), Water Treatment 2 (WT 2); reduced to once in 15 days and the Control, watering depended upon moisture availability in the soil.

Table 1. Developmental patterns in the leaves of water stressed and unstressed soybean plants measured immediately after the termination of the water deficit stress experiment.

Soybean genotypes	Mean plant height (cm)		Mean no. of branches		Flowering plants (%)		Mean no. of pods produced		Survival frequency (%)	
	TP 1	TP 2	TP 1	TP 2	TP 1	TP 2	TP 1	TP 2	TP 1	TP 2
Dundee	25.2[a]	24.1[a]	3.0[a]	3.0[a]	—	—	—	—	—	—
LS 678	40.0[b]	26.4[b]	3.0[a]	3.0[a]	—	—	—	—	—	—
LS 677	33.3[c]	26.5[b]	4.0[b]	3.0[a]	1.00[a]	—	7.0[a]	—	15.0[a]	—
Peking	24.2[d]	23.5[a]	4.0[b]	2.0[b]	15.0[b]	—	3.0[b]	—	30.0[b]	—
TGx 1740-2F	27.3[e]	21.0[c]	2.0[c]	3.0[a]	—	—	—	—	—	—
TGx 1835-10E	26.1[f]	20.7[d]	3.0[a]	3.0[a]	—	—	—	—	—	—

Percentage survival frequency was calculated from the number of plants/ genotype that survive until the termination of the water stress deficit experiment.

Statistical significance among the values is designated by different superscript letters. Values within columns showing different letters are statistically varied (at 0.05) by ANOVA.

Table 2. Vegetative growth and flowering response of soybean plants subjected to water deficit stress conditions.

were observed. Soybean cultivar LS 677 and Peking showed some resistance with 15 and 30% survival rate (**Table 2**). A few plants in these two genotypes exhibited moderate stress effects among all the cultivars assessed. There were no differences in the lengths of root system and shoots observed in water stress resistant cultivars (LS 677 and Peking) in comparison with those severely affected (Dundee, LS 678, TGx 1740-2F and TGx 1835-10E) in both WT 1 and WT 2 plants.

Klamkowski and Treder [21] reported almost similar results in water stressed strawberry plants. In addition, there were no major differences, especially in root lengths that were observed between water stressed plants and the control. The report cited inhibition of growth by water stressed plants, involving decrease in root expansion as suggested by Boyer [22]. This claim probably led to the observed root phenotype in water stressed strawberry plants. This is in contrast with finding in this study and most of the other suggestions made on root phenotypes during water stress. In general, root formation has been found to increase in length during water stress, with roots growing deep into the soil in search for moisture [17, 19, 23, 24]. This further development in the root system is an attempt by plants to increase the uptake of water in order to sustain growth as observed in this study.

3.2. Anatomical changes in response to water stress

The WT 1 and WT 2 plants demonstrated a different internal anatomy compared to the control plants. Stem cortex of water stressed plant were generally smaller compared to the cortex in stems of plants in the control (**Figure 2**). However, vascular tissue thickening and expansion was observed in both the roots and stems of water stressed and control plants. The development of the secondary tissues in water stressed plants, especially the deposition of secondary xylem cells (as viewed in **Figure 2a, b**), was interrupted by the gradual rapturing of the pith which resulted in the formation of pith canals. Pith canals are hollow centres, called central canals, which are usually formed in woody shrubs and trees. They are formed when the earliest vascular tissues, protoxylem, is destroyed by the formation of new metaxylem as the root or stem grows in diameter. In gymnosperms, these canals are instead used by the pine trees to store resin and they are more associated with the cortical tissue of the stems than the pith [25]. In stems of plants such as seedless vascular plants (horsetails), these canals are naturally formed to reduce the weight of the stem thus, increasing stem strength and resistance to buckling [18]. However, the formation of canals (breaking down of the soybean pith tissue) observed in roots and stems may have resulted from water stress. Furthermore, this may have possibly impacted negatively on the growth of plants, particularly when induced as a result of severe water stress, like in WT 2.

Even though the pith is poor in nutrients [26], the parenchyma cells can still function in storage of nutrients and water for the plant. Pallardy [27] suggested that, rapturing could also destroy the interconnectivity between the storage parenchyma of the pith with the cortex, disrupting short distance transport that occurs through the rays via secondary xylem. The variations in canal diameters between WT 1 and WT 2 (**Figure 2a**, **b**, including canal in the root- **d**) may be in response to the different water stress regimes or the genotype variability of the soybeans used. Canal diameters in soybean WT 2 plants were larger than the diameter observed in WT 1 plants (**Figure 2a**, **b**). Soybean cultivar LS 677 and LS 678 showed little resistance to the rapturing of the pith, compared to cultivar Peking and Dundee. This was the case, even though cultivar LS 677 and Peking were the only varieties more resistant to water stress treatment (WT 1). This could be both a genetically-linked response and the reaction or effects of water stress conditions to the tissue development. In cultivar Peking, TGx 1740-2F and TGx 1835-10E, pith canals appeared to be continuously cut from the central pith further to the cortical cells. This induced complete disruption of water transportation through some part of the xylems, xylem rays and nutrient transport by the phloem tissues. The cutting of water supply may have resulted in the poor survival rates observed in most of the cultivars (**Table 2**). But, the absence of pith canals in stems of the control plants furthermore suggests a relationship between water deficit and the change in anatomy of the soybean plants. When the imposed environmental stress reduced the rate of tissue development, the length of xylem rays in roots was also reduced.

The reduction occurred when growth is affected by death of tissues and slowing down of metabolism as a result of the stress. Alteration in plant metabolism affect cell division, thus cell elongation and expansion is negatively affected as evidenced in **Figure 2d**, **e**). The xylem cell portion in the roots of water stressed plants was reduced compared to xylem tissue diameter in the control. Yamaguchi and Sharp [28] indicated that, water stress induce changes in root growth and cell length distribution which may be directly related to growth inhibition in roots, especially at root elongation zones. Another example is by Schuppler et al. [6] who also indicated the reduction on mitotic activity of mesophyll tissues in wheat (*Triticum aestivum*) seedlings subjected to mild water deficit. These reports indicate that, the lack of adequate water supply decreases the rate of cell division and tissue expansion in all plant organs, although root morphology may appear less affected in contrast to root anatomy. Munns and Sharp [29] made similar remarks following their investigation on the effect of abscisic acid (ABA) on shoot and root growths during salinity and drought stress.

4. Effect of water deficit on plant metabolism

The synthesis and breakdown of metabolites to yield energy is required for the many activities that plants depend upon. But, when plants are exposed to drought stress conditions, physiological and metabolic changes occur. Immediate acclimatisation by the alteration of plant morphology is therefore required for plants to be adapted to the changing environments. Whether plants succeed to acclimatise or not, the subsequent phenotypic modifications observed in water stressed plants would be a function of the metabolic changes. In soybean, like other leguminous plants, decrease in the leaf area, number of individual leaves and the total number of branches per plant is normally observed [16, 24]. However, on the metabolic section, water stressed plants experiences a dramatic decrease in photosynthetic rates as a consequence of the modification in photosynthetic structures and chloroplastidic pigments. Chloroplastidic pigments involve all plant pigments such as chlorophylls and carotenoid pigments embedded in the thylakoid membranes of parenchyma mesophylls [18]. These pigments are primary molecules responsible for making sure that light energy from the sun is captured and converted to chemical energy required for metabolism.

This is the main route in which energy used for synthesis of biological products enters our biosphere. Water stress adversely limits this process by inhibiting the functioning of structure serving as primary support for photosynthetic metabolism. According to Kwon and Woo [24] drought reduce photosynthesis by limiting stomatal operations. In line with this report, the soybean plants subjected to water stress (WT 1 and WT 2) kept their stomata closed to reduce transpiration, hence trying to preserve water. The stomatal micrograph in **Figure 3** illustrates closed stomatal apertures (c, d) prepared from leaves collected during the day. The closure of stomata in turn reduces the concentration of CO_2 required in the mesophyll for carboxylation process during the manufacturing of photosynthates. This phenomenon was also reported by Dekov et al. [31], Evert and Eichhorn [18], Lopez-Carbonell et al. [30] and Taiz et al. [17]. Additionally, there were significant variations in stomatal density exhibited by the different genotypes.

Water stressed soybean cultivar TGx 1740-2F and LS 677 exhibited low density of stomata with an average of 154 and 106 in WT 1 and WT 2 respectively, among all the cultivars used (**Table 1**). Furthermore, the two TGx cultivars (TGx 1740-2F and TGx 1835-10E) did not show extensive variations in the stomata among all water stressed plants, including the control. The mean leaf areas of the water stressed plants were also significantly lower compared to the control. The decrease in the leaf area of the plants posed negative effects on the rate of photosynthesis by reducing the leaf surface area in which light is captured. Anatomically, water stress also had an effect on leaf mesophyll thickness which also had an impact on photosynthesis. Cramer and Browman [32] attributed this to the changes in the rate of cellular expansion, which was observed in the maize mesophyll tissues when cell division and differentiation appeared affected by drought stress. However, plants growing in soil grounds of very lower water potential possess poor cell formation and expansion. Schuppler et al. [6] also reported this when assessing the effects of water stress on rate of cell division or mitotic activity on wheat leaf tissues. The report indicated that generally, leaf tissue expansion rate is reduced to more than 50% when plants are subjected to drought stress. In terms of physiological response to water stress, the reduction in chlorophyll content index (CCI) in water stressed plants was

http://dx.doi.org/10.5772/intechopen.72899

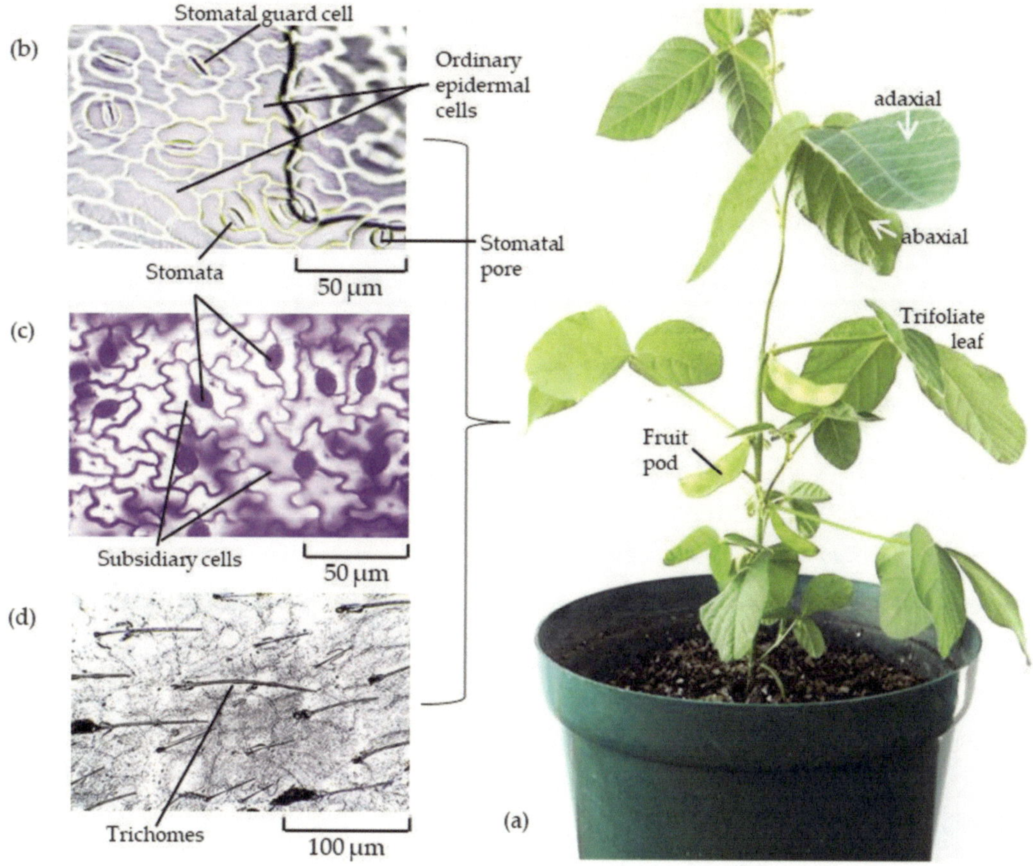

Figure 3. Dermal tissue of the leaf of a typical soybean plant. (a) Soybean plant at R4 stage. (b) Field of epidermal cells of a soybean plant. (c) Light micrograph of slightly higher magnification of stomatal complexes on a soybean leaf. (d) Light micrograph in the epidermis showing epidermal hairs.

recorded, and the decreases in chlorophyll contents varied according to imposed water stress treatments (**Figure 4**). Plant irrigated once in 15 days (WT 2) showed remarkable decrease in CCI (**Figure 4d**) than WT 1 plants (**Figure 4b**).

Control plants did not exhibit significant reduction in CCI nor variation in all cultivars' CCI measurements even before when water treatments were imposed on water stressed plants (**Figure 4a, b**). But then, differences were not expected in the CCI estimates of control plants measured early during growth and later before termination of the experiment, since the plants were adequately watered. Therefore, as expected the chlorophyll degradation was not induced on control plants as a result of water stress. As the differences in the chlorophyll content and degradation were observed in water stressed plants, these findings were in line with Dhanda et al. [33] and Benjamin and Nielsen [34]'s reports on the effects of drought on plant metabolism. As indicated on Section 2, to examine and confirm the degradation of chlorophyll and its subsequent effects on photosynthetic activity, starch analysis was performed. Leaves detached from randomly selected soybean plants were obtained and taken to the laboratory for starch analysis. The leaves were bleached in boiling 90% ethanol and incubated in dilute iodine (0.5 M) solution (2:1) for 3 minutes and then rinsed with distilled water. Rinsing is necessary to remove excess iodine solution

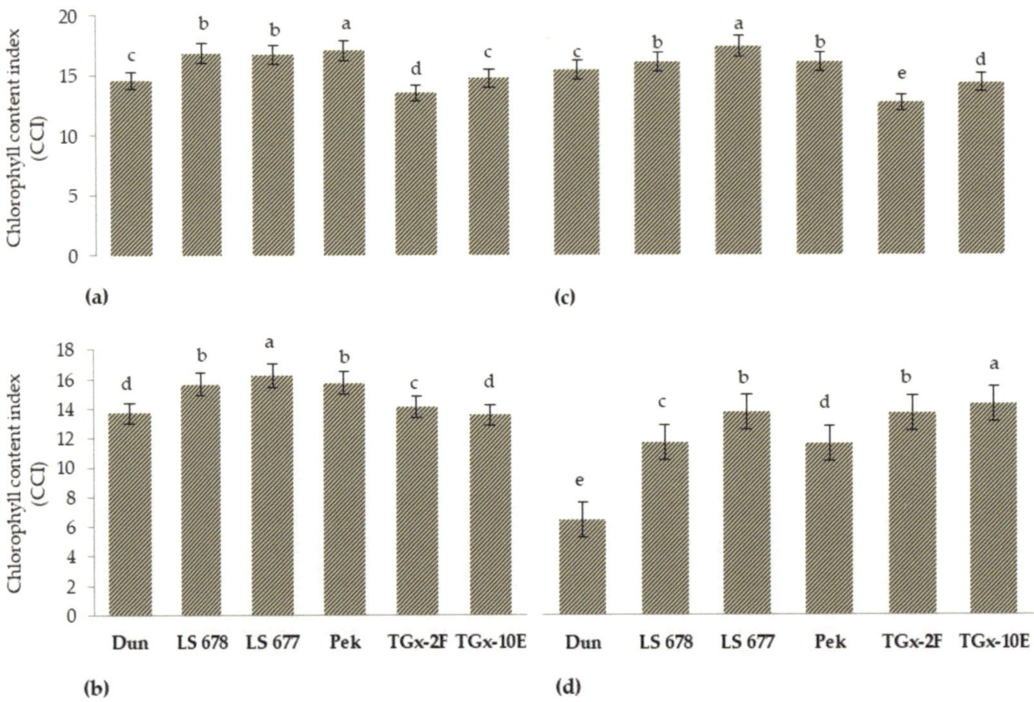

Figure 4. Effect of water deficit stress on photosynthetic pigment (chlorophyll) content of soybean plants expressed to CCI. (a) Chlorophyll content of control plants during early growth stages (V3). (b) Leaf chlorophyll content of the control during early reproductive stages. (c) Amount of chlorophyll content in WT 1 plants. (d) Leaf chlorophyll content in WT 2. Data represent CCI means and the different letters denote significant differences of the means at $p < 0.05$.

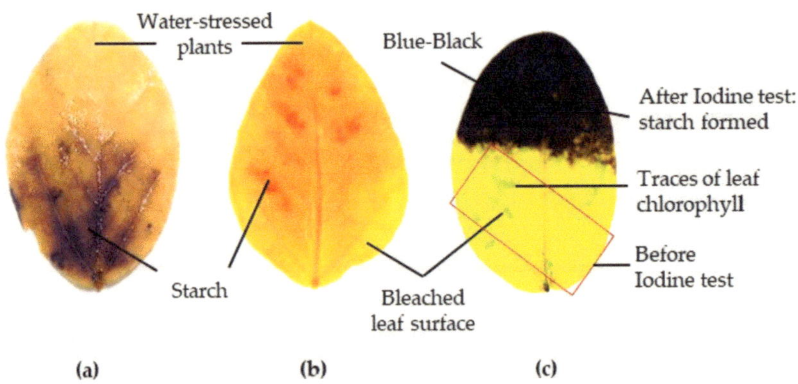

Figure 5. Iodine test on ethanol bleached leaves. After bleaching and staining with iodine: (a) Show traces of starch on leaflet taken from water stress plants (WT 1). (b) Absence of or minor starch traces on severely water stressed leaflet (WT 2). (c) Starch content (blue black colour) on leaflet taken from the control plants.

on the leaves while a colour change occurs. The iodine stained leaves (**Figure 5a–c**) were then visualised under a ZIESS Discovery V12 stereo microscope mounted with an ICc5 Axio-Camera. The presence of high starch content was observed in the control (**Figure 5c**); whereby starch contents in WT 1 (**Figure 5a**) and WT 2 (**Figure 5b**) were very drastically reduced because of poor photosynthetic activity. Intense blue-black colour on the leaves of control plants indicate the presence of starch, generated from the photosynthesised carbohydrates. Only minor traces of starch were observed from WT 1 and WT 2 leaves due to water stress.

5. Nodulation

The formation of cell protuberance containing nitrogen-fixing Gram-negative bacteria in the roots of legumes plays an important role in improving plant growth characteristics, crop productivity and maintaining soil fertility. This establishment of lumps on roots of plants (known as nodulation) guarantees the supply of fixed atmospheric N_2 for use in the synthesis of proteins, nucleic acids and other necessary nitrogen-containing compounds required for plant, animal and human growth and development. However, various reports have indicated that, water stress induces low frequencies of nodulation in many legumes, including soybean. Miao et al. [35] provided evidence that verifies sensitivity of soybean nodulating root cells and Rhizobium to water stress. In 2003, Ramos et al. [36] also indicated that, water stress affect nodulation in other legume species like *Phaseolus vulgaris* L. Failure for soybean roots to produce effective nodulations affect the metabolism of nitrogenous and carbonic compounds in the plant. The changes resulting into decreased nodulation could cause reduction in various aspects of plant growth (stem height, stem wood diameter and root dry weight) due to drought as reported by Shetta [37]. Additionally, Shetta indicated that the initiated nodules can become thickened and more resistant to infection by *Rhizobium* as a result of this stress. Poor nodulation can be induced by poor plant nutrition, seed filling, or abiotic stress factors. In WT 2 plants, where irrigation was withheld for 15 days, nodulation was severely affected (**Figure 6f**). It was found that nodules stopped fixing nitrogen and then started decomposing. Nodulation and nitrogen fixation in the WT 1 also decreased following imposed water deficit stress. The nodules turned green (**Figure 6e**) and this predominant green colour indicated inefficient fixation by Rhizobium strain in contrast to highly efficient red-pinkish nodules in the control (**Figure 6d**). This inefficiency may have been caused by the poor amounts of assimilates that are exchanged from soybeans to the bacteria due to reduced rates of photosynthesis in the leaves. Plants do not get fixed nitrogen from Rhizobium for free. For plants to receive fixed atmospheric nitrogen, in a form that is directly available for growth (nitrates–NO_3^- and ammonium–NH_4^+), plants must give bacteria sugars. This symbiotic relationship was reported by Dupont et al. [38], Serraj et al. [39] and Stajkovic et al. [40] as the major stimulant of increased plant biomass, stabilising atmospheric CO_2 by stabilising C–N ratio. The symbiosis establishment is playing a very critical role in ecological and agronomic supply of N_2, estimated to account for a total of about 65% of the nitrogen fixed in legumes used for agriculture globally.

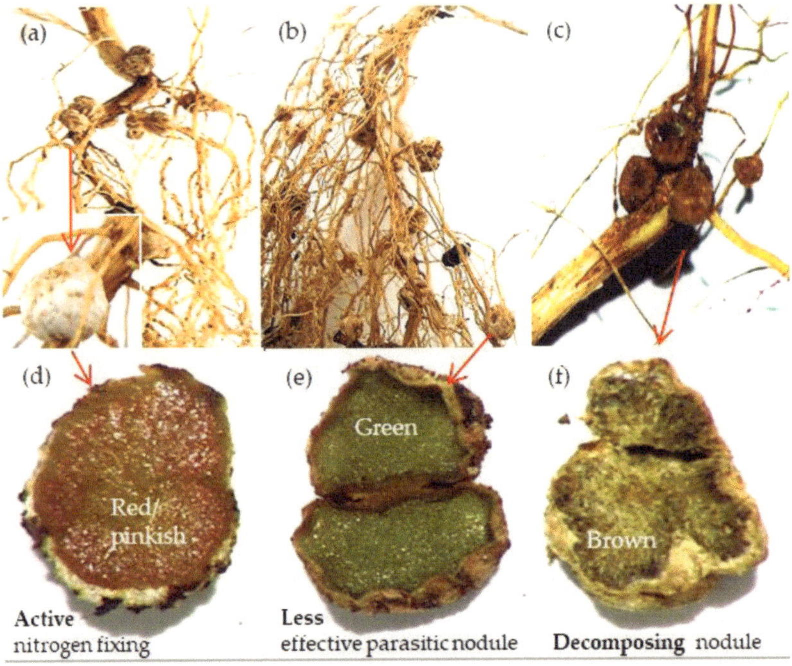

Figure 6. Soybean plants with nodulated roots. (a) Healthy nodules on soybean control plants. (b) Roots of WT 1 with numerous mature nodule structures. (c) WT 2 stressed plant root showing poor nodulation. (d) Nitrogen (N) fixing nodules with *Rhizobia* as observed in the control. (e) Less effective nodules from WT 1 roots. (f) Decomposing root nodule of WT 2 plants.

6. Impact of water deficit on flowering and fruiting

The soybean genotypes showed great differences in the percentage flowering, pod formation and other yield related components. Water stressed plants produced less than 2% yield, in the two soybean cultivars (LS 677 and Peking) that survived induced water stress. A few WT 1 plants subjected to water stress continued their growth until flowering and pod formation stages. However, flower and fruit pod abortions were simultaneously observed leading to 7.0 and 3.0 mean pod number observed in the few plants that had survived (**Table 3**). These numbers were not comparable with the yield component data recorded for these cultivars in the control. Soriano et al. [41] determined a positive relationship between yield quantity by estimating grain number and weight in early planted sunflower by timing induction of environment stress. In line with this report, positive yield characteristics that include; total percentage of flowering plants, mean number of pods and average pod length, pod weight and seed weight (per 100 seeds) were observed in all of the cultivars in the control. In contrast, as a result of water stress, a significant number of flower abortions (10–15%) were observed in cultivar Dundee, LS 677, TGx 1740-2F and TGx 1835-10E which showed the least survival rate at 0%.

The variation observed in control plants however, did not seem to affect pod development and maturation, thus, could be attributed to the genotype performance than the environmental

Soybean genotypes	Mean plant height (cm)	Mean no. of branches	No. of flowering plants (%)	Mean no. of pods produced	Survival frequency (%)
Dundee	31.0[a]	6.0[a]	80.0[a]	21.0[a]	80.0[a]
LS 678	41.0[b]	5.0[b]	95.0[b]	32.0[b]	95.0[b]
LS 677	49.1[c]	6.0[a]	100.0[c]	36.0[c]	100.0[c]
Peking	51.0[d]	6.0[a]	100.0[c]	29.0[d]	100.0[c]
TGx 1740-2F	47.1[e]	5.0[b]	95.0[b]	19.0[e]	95.0[b]
TGx 1835-10E	49.5[c]	6.0[a]	100.0[c]	21.0[a]	100.0[c]
Additional data on yield and yield components of untreated soybean plants					
	Ave. pod length (cm)	Ave. pod weight (g)	Seed weight/100 seeds (g)		
Dundee	4.06[a]	0.44[a]	18.53[a]		
LS 678	3.38[b]	0.49[b]	14.06[b]		
LS 677	5.23[c]	0.50[c]	14.02[b]		
Peking	3.96[d]	0.38[d]	9.54[c]		
TGx 1740-2F	3.40[b]	0.51[c]	12.03[d]		
TGx 1835-10E	3.94[d]	0.49[b]	12.87[e]		

Plant watering was carried out depending on the moisture availability in the soil. Data on yield components was recorded on the day that the experiment was terminated.

The mean number of pods produced was determined 2 weeks after the pods were successfully produced in order to avoid counting fruit pods that will eventually not produce seeds. Data represent the means and values followed by different letters are significantly different (in columns) (at $p \leq 0.05$) by ANOVA.

Table 3. Vegetative growth and flowering response of soybean plants subjected to normal water conditions.

growth conditions (**Table 3**). In the control, a single genotypic setback was observed in cultivar TGx 1740-2F and TGx 1835-10E, which were the only ones producing the lowest number of pods, respectively. The effect of water stress in other oilseed grains such as sunflower, common bean, wheat, barley and maize were reported [41–43]. According to Jaleel et al. [19] the changes in the photosynthetic pigments and the decrease in metabolic functioning of the plant lead to decreased yield productivity. Seed yield and seed's morphological characters can also be affected by drought [44]. In cultivar Peking, the interaction between water deficit stress and seed appearance resulting from the genotype was not severely pronounced. The seeds appeared intensely shrinked and decreased in seed size due to loss of seed moisture, immediately after harvesting. This response was observed in another study assessing seed longevity in soybean seeds (data not published), clearly suggesting this as a dormancy or viability mechanism compared to other genotypes. In general, significant differences were observed during flowering, pod formation and seed maturation/ filling, as well as in the seed phenotypic characteristics among all cultivars in the control. Many water stressed plants (WT 1 and WT 2) did not survive to reach flowering as observed in the normally irrigated plants of the control (**Tables 2** and **3**).

7. Other biotic and abiotic stress effects

Plants are normally adapted to grow in complex and diverse environments. The success in growth establishment, reproduction and productivity of plant species rely upon a set of environmental conditions, natural resources and the interactions (beneficial or harmful) that exist among plants and other organisms. However, certain types of interactions, especially those including biological factors such as insects, parasites, viruses and bacterial pathogens have detrimental effects on plants. In addition, the non-living physical or chemical factors such as light, temperature, salinity, water, nutrient and other variables that can be found in the aquatic or terrestrial ecosystem also have major impacts on plant life. All above-mentioned factors may induce plant stress, defined by Taiz et al. [17] as a condition that prevent a given plant from achieving its maximum growth and reproductive potential as measured by vegetative growth, flowering, seed formation and yield quantity. Gerhardson [45] gave further information by providing more insights on disease symptoms caused by pathogenic strains of *Fusarium*, *Cylindrocarpon*, *Phoma* and *Pythium* mostly on legume crops. Strains of the genera *Pythium* have also been found to cause seedling mortality in cowpea [46]. These soil-borne legume pathogens, including other wide spread disease causing fungi; induce root, stem and leaf rots in pea, beans and alfalfa [45]. Abiotic environmental stress dramatically affects growth and productivity of many cereals, oilseeds, vegetables and fruit crops.

Oilseeds such as soybeans have suffered major losses from the short and prolonged occurrence of abiotic stress, especially drought, extreme temperatures, flooding and waterlogging [47]. Plants experiencing drought stress may also endure other stress effects simultaneously, like salinity and heat stress. Multiple stress effects and symptoms may be concomitantly induced by the occurrence of a single stress as described by Miransari [48] leading to combinational abiotic stress. In soybean, drought stress has many negative consequences ranging from reduced production of signalling and communication metabolites, decreased photosynthetic assimilates, nutrient deficiency, accumulation of reactive oxygen species (ROS) and reduction in nitrogen (N) fixation by affecting symbiotic relationship with *Rhizobium* species [49–52]. Soybean is an important crop for the production of oils and proteins used for feed and human consumption. It is a potential source for biodiesel and has been used to manufacture a number of pharmaceutical products [53]. But, the high sensitivity to water deficit stress shown in this study by this crop encourage the development of stress tolerant soybean varieties. Drought and other growth constraints are inevitable consequences of climate change. Therefore, investigation on the physiological, anatomical and morphological response of soybean to these biotic and abiotic constraints is highly recommended.

8. Water stress management and crop improvement

As previously discussed, drought stress is the most widely known and devastating stress factor that limit plant growth, development and productivity. Khaine and Woo [54] reported that, frequent drought effects recently and currently experienced, are largely induced by the changes in climatic conditions. The continuously fluctuating meteorological conditions in many regions worldwide have led to tremendous adversities on agriculture, biodiversity, wildlife and subsequently, the well-beings of many people. Plants normally evolve in order to adapt and adjust to the low water conditions or any other biotic and abiotic constraint. These adaptive measures are an important event of evolution in the history of life, with far reaching consequences as described by Kenrick and Crane [55]. However, this is a very slow process in nature, even if it may result in greater diversity of plants, making changes in plants at their physiological, biochemical and molecular levels. These changes show a wide range of adaptations, at different levels in which plants attempt to deal with drought stress [56]. Plants manage water stress in various ways. They regulate stomatal closure to reduce water loss, especially through transpiration. The stomatal opening and closing is very essential for gaseous exchange as reported by Osakabe et al. [57]. They are controlled by complex regulatory events mediated by abscisic acid (ABA) signalling and ion transport induced by abiotic stress. Nonetheless, stomata closure negatively affects the rates of photosynthetic metabolism by lowering the amount of CO_2. Plants also alter metabolic functions in order to inhibit the production of reactive oxygen species (ROS) such as superoxide (O_2^-), and H_2O_2 [52, 58]. Other changes involve development of strategies to fix CO_2 with minimum loss of water. For example; many C_3 plants do not have photosynthetic adaptations to reduce the loss of CO_2 molecules by separating photorespiration from the Calvin cycle. However, some succulent plants use Crassulaceae acid metabolism (CAM) to salvage CO_2 minimising photorespiration thus, saving water.

In monocots such as maize and wheat, CO_2 is fixed in the mesophyll spongy cells (a light-dependent process) and in the specialised cell around the leaf veins called the bundle sheath (light-independent). These monocotyledonous plants are referred to as C_4 plants and they produce oxaloacetate which is converted into malate, transported into the bundle sheath for use in Calvin cycle [17, 59, 60]. Both C_4 and CAM plants are well adapted to hot, dry environments than the C_3 plants like peanut (*Arachis hypogaea*), potato (*Solanum tuberosum*) and soybean (*Glycine max* L.). These C_3 plants lack strategies to efficiently and effectively manage water use. In addition to all of the metabolic strategies mentioned above, modern genetic engineering technology can be used. This technology is focused on breeding biotic/ abiotic stress tolerant plants. The biotechnological approaches such as *Agrobacterium*-mediated genetic transformation allow manipulation of the host plant's genome for the expression of foreign genes required in the plant stress response. This technique was initially used to isolate genes used for stress tolerance in *Arabidopsis*. This plant was only used as a model plant and has played an important role in elucidating the basic processes constituting the expression of regulatory genes for stress tolerance [61]. The insights from research on *Arabidopsis* have been used in attempts of unravelling biotic/ abiotic stress effects in plants, subsequently resulting in the development of transgenic plants tolerant to drought, salinity and chilling stress. Montero-Tavera et al. [62] reported upregulation of a number of genes in two common bean varieties with different susceptibility to drought stress. Variety Pinto Villa was relatively susceptible than cultivar Carioca. The reports indicated that drought tolerant variety displayed a more developed root vascular tissue system under stress conditions, when compared to the other non-transgenic cultivars. Differential root phenotype showing variations in root lengths, surface area and fineness of the root system was also reported by Abenavoli et al. [63]. In soybean, stress tolerant genes were introduced and DREB or ARED genes expressed to show improved tolerance to water stress under greenhouse conditions [11, 64]. The genetic transformation of many crops, including soybean via *in vitro* or *in vivo* transformation techniques is still very difficult to achieve, despite the aforementioned successes. Several drought tolerant cultivars have been reported in rice (*Oryza sativa*), maize (*Zea mays* L.) and kidney bean (*Phaseolus vulgaris* L.) by Liu et al. [65], Saijo et al. [66] and Shou et al. [67]. The methods used for genetic transformation of these crops are continuously optimised to establish efficient and reproducible protocols using *Agrobacterium tumefaciens*. Lastly, agronomic practices such as reduction of water loss from irrigation systems, minimising water inputs and increasing crop water use efficiency can also be employed to manage water stress [68].

9. Conclusions and perspectives

This study revealed that soybeans are primarily affected by water deficit. Cultivars highly susceptible to water stress were easily distinguishable from those showing mild stress effects on the basis of the morphological and anatomical characters in stems, leaves and roots. Morphological architecture, anatomical features and chloroplastidic pigments were significantly affected by the induced water stress. This comprehensive insights regarding the internal and external growth characteristics including, aspects that involve the physiological processes is crucial for the pursuit of genetically modified plants. Soybean remains one of the most important oilseeds that are commercially and subsistently cultivated worldwide. The crop contains higher amounts of proteins, oils, fibre and minerals required for poultry feedstocks and human consumption. As a result of this, the elite superior genotypes of this crop still need to be investigated in order to identify the cultivars that would serve as genetic resource for breeding or genetic engineering, ultimately providing cultivars to be used for agricultural purposes showing high tolerance to abiotic stress, especially drought.

Acknowledgements

This study was carried out with the support by the Department of Biodiversity, University of Limpopo. The author acknowledges Dr. P.W. Mokwala and Mr. F. Nndwambi for providing seeds of soybean. Many thanks to Mr. L. Ramoba, F. Nukeri, S. Thosago, F.M. Masiya, R. Mudau, V.L. Makwana, L.R. Mahuluhulu, L.M. Marotola, K.K. Boshomane, M. Lutombo and T. Maleka for their technical support.

Author details

Phetole Mangena

Address all correspondence to: mangena.phetole@gmail.com

Department of Biodiversity, School of Molecular and Life Sciences, Faculty of Science and Agriculture, University of Limpopo, Sovenga, South Africa

References

[1] Mattson JW, Haack RA. The role of drought in outbreak of plant eating insects. Bioscience. 1987;**37**(2):110-118

[2] Wrather A, Koenning S. Effects of diseases on soybean yields in the United States 1996 to 2007. Plant Management Network. 2009;**401**(01):1-7

[3] Liu S, Yan D, Wang J, Wang B, Wang G, Yang M. Drought mitigation ability index and application based on balance between water supply and demand. Water. 2015;**7**:1792-1807

[4] Petit JR, Jouzel J, Raynaud D, Barkov NI, Barnola JM, Basile I, Bender M, Chappellaz J, Davis J, Delayque G, Delmolte M, Kotlyakov VM, Legrand M, Lipenkov V, Lorius C, Pepin L, Ritz C, Saltzman E, Stievenard M. Climate and atmospheric history of the past 420,000 years from the Vostok ice Core Antarctica. Nature. 1999;**399**:429-436

[5] Shao HB, Chu LY, Jaleel CA, Zhao CX. Water-deficit stress-induced anatomical changes in higher plants. Comptes Rendus Biologies. 2008;**331**:215-225

[6] Schuppler U, He PH, John PCL, Munns R. Effect of water stress on cell division and cell-division-cycle 2-like cell-cycle kinase activity in wheat leaves. Plant Physiology. 1998;**177**:667-678

[7] Jewell MC, Campbell BC, Godwin ID. Transgenic plants for abiotic stress resistance. In: Kole C, Michler C, Abbott AG, Hall TC, editors. Transgenic Crop Plants: Volume 1; Principles and Development. Berlin Heidelberg: Springer-Verlag; 2010. pp. 76-132

[8] Lisar SYS, Motafakkerazad R, Hossain MM, Rahman IMM. Water stress in plants: Causes, effects and responses. In: Rahman MM, Hasegawa H, editors. Water Stress. Rijeka, Croatia: InTech Open; 2012

[9] Food, Agriculture and Natural Resources (FANR). 2017. Food security; early warning system. Directorate for the Southern African Development Community (SADC). Issue no. 3

[10] Food and Agriculture Organization of the United Nations (FAO). 2015. Monitoring agriculture drought with remote sensing data. FAO Agriculture Stress Index System

[11] Ishaq MN, Ehirim BO. Improving soybean productivity using biotechnology approach in Nigeria. World Journal of Agriculture Sciences. 2014;**2**(2):13-18

[12] Cornelissen JHC, Lavorel S, Garnier E, Diaz S, Buchmann N, Gurvisch DE, Reich PB, Steege H, Morgan HD, van der Heijden MGA, Pausa JG, Poorter H. A handbook of protocols for standardized and easy measurements of plant functional traits worldwide. Australian Journal of Botany. 2003;**51**:335-380

[13] Yeung EC. A Beginner's Guide to the Study of Plant Structure. Calgary Alberta, Canada: Association for Biology Laboratory Education (ABLE); 1998. pp. 125-136

[14] Richter GL, Junior AZ, Streck NA, Guedes JVC, Kraulich B, Da-Rocha TSM, Winck JEM, Cera JC. Estimating leaf area of modern soybean cultivars by a non-destructive method. Crop Production and Management. 2014;**74**(4):476-425

[15] North Dakota State University (NDSU). Soybean Growth and Management: Quick Guide. Fargo, North Dakota: NDSU Agriculture Extension Service; 2015

[16] Mabulwana PT. Determination of drought stress tolerance among soybean varieties using morphological and physiological markers. Masters' Dissertation. Sovenga, South Africa: University of Limpopo; 2013

[17] Taiz L, Zeiger E, Moller IM, Murphy A. Plant Physiology and Development. 6th ed. USA: Sinauer Associates; 2015. p. 561

[18] Evert RF, Eichhorn SE. Raven Biology of Plants. 8th ed. New York: W.H. Freeman and Company; 2013. pp. 541-547

[19] Jaleel CA, Manivannan P, Wahid A, Farooq M, Al-Juburi HJ, Somasundararam R, Panneerselvam R. Drought stress in plants: A review on morphological characteristics and pigments composition. International Journal of Agriculture and Biology. 2009;**11**: 100-105

[20] Nosalewicz A, Lipiec J. The effect of compacted soil layers on vertical root distribution and water uptake by wheat. Plant and Soil. 2013;**375**:229-240

[21] Klamkowski K, Treder W. Morphological and physiological responses of strawberry plants to water stress. Agriculturae Conspectus Scientificus. 2006;**71**(4):159-165

[22] Boyer JS. Leaf enlargement and metabolic rates in corn, soybean and sunflower at various leaf water potentials. Plant Physiology. 1970;**46**:233-235

[23] Fenta BA, Beebe SE, Kunert KJ, Burridge JD, Barlow KM, Lynch JP, Foyer CH. Field phenotyping of soybean roots for drought stress tolerance. Agronomy. 2014;**4**:418-435

[24] Kwon MY, Woo SY. Plant's responses to drought and shade environments. African Journal of Biotechnology. 2016;**15**(2):29-31

[25] Rosner S, Hannrup B. Resin canal traits relevant for constitutive resistance of Norway spruce against bark beetles: Environmental and genetic variability. Forest Ecology and Management. 2004;**200**:77-78

[26] Kirkendall LR, Biedermann PHW, Jordal BH. Evolution and diversity of bark and ambrosia bettles. In: Vega FE, editor. Bark Beetles: Biology and Ecology of Native and Invasive Species. USA: Academic Press; 2015. pp. 85-156

[27] Pallardy SG. Vegetative growth. In: Physiology of Woody Plants. 3rd ed. USA: Academic Press; 2008. pp. 39-86

[28] Yamaguchi M, Sharp RE. Complexity and coordination of root growth at low water potential: Recent advances from transcriptomic and proteomic analyses. Plant, Cell & Environment. 2010;**33**:590-603

[29] Munns R, Sharp RE. Involvement of abscisic acid in controlling plant growth in soil of low water potential. Australian Journal of Plant Physiology. 1993;**20**(5):425-437

[30] Lopez-Carbonell M, Alegre L, Vanonckelen H. Effect of water stress on cellular ultrastructure and on concentration of endogenous abscisic acid and indole-3-acetic acid in *Fatsia jabonica* leaves. Plant Growth Regulation. 1994;**14**:29-35

[31] Dekov I, Tsonev T, Yordanov I. Effect of water stress and high-temperature stress on the structure and activity of photosynthetic apparatus of *Zea mays* and *Helianthus annuus*. Photosynthetica. 2000;**38**:361-366

[32] Cramer GR, Browman DC. Kinetics of maize leaf elongation: I. Increased yield threshold limits short-term, steady-state elongation rates after exposure to salinity. Journal of Experimental Botany. 1991;**42**:1417-1426

[33] Dhanda SS, Sethi GS, Behl RK. Indices of drought tolerance in wheat genotypes at early stages of plant growth. Journal of Agricultural Crop Science. 2004;**190**:6-12

[34] Benjamin JG, Nielsen DC. Water deficit effects on root distribution of soybean, field pea and chickpea. Field Crops Research. 2006;**97**:248-253

[35] Miao S, Jin J, Shi H, Wang G. Effect of short-term drought and flooding on soybean nodulation and yield at key nodulation stages under pot culture. Journal of Food, Agriculture and Environment. 2012;**10**(3):819-824

[36] Ramos MLG, Persons R, Sprent JI, James EK. Effect of water stress on nitrogen fixation and nodule structure of common bean. Pesquisa Agropecuária Brasileira. 2003;**38**(3):339-347

[37] Shetta ND. Influence of drought stress on growth and nodulation of *Acacia origena* (Hunde) inoculated with indigenous rhizobium isolated from Saudi Arabia. American-Eurasian Journal of Agricultural and Environmental Sciences. 2015;**15**(5):699-706

[38] Dupont L, Alloing G, Pierre O, Elmsehli S, Hopkins J, Herouart D, Frendo P. The legume root nodule from symbiotic nitrogen fixation to senescence. In: Nayata T, editor. Senescence. Rijeka, Croatia: InTech Open; 2012. pp. 137-168

[39] Serraj R, Sinclair TR, Allen LH. Soybean nodulation and N_2 fixation response to drought under carbon dioxide enrichment. Plant, Cell and Environment. 1998;**21**:491-500

[40] Stajkovic O, Delic D, Josic D, Kuzmanovic D, Rasulic N, Knezevic-Vukcevic J. Improvement of common bean growth by co-inoculation with *Rhizobium* and plant growth-promoting bacteria. Romanian Biotechnological Letters. 2011;**16**(1):5919-5926

[41] Soriano MA, Villalobos FJ, Feres E. Stress timing effects on sunflower harvest index. In: Villalobos FJ, Testi L, editors. European Society for Agronomy, VII ESA Congress 15-18 July, Spain Book of Proceedings, 2002:142-143

[42] Edward D, Wright D. The effects of winter water-logging and summer drought on the growth and yield of winter wheat (*Triticum aestivum* L.). European Journal of Agronomy. 2008;**28**:234-244

[43] Lipiec J, Doussan C, Nosalewicz A, Kondracka K. Effect of drought and heat stress on plant growth and yield: A review. International Agrophysics. 2013;**27**:463-477

[44] Sepanlo N, Talebi R, Rokhzadi A, Mohammadi H. Morphological and physiological behaviour in soybean (*Glycine max*) genotypes to drought stress implemented at pre- and post- anthesis stages. Acta Biologica Szegediensis. 2014;**58**(2):109-113

[45] Gerhardson JL. Pathogenicity of clover root pathogens to pea, bean and lucerne. Journal of Plant Disease and Protection. 2002;**109**(2):142-151

[46] Suleiman MN. Occurrence of *Pythium aphanidermatum* on cowpea (*Vigna unguiculata* (L.) Walp) in Nigeria. Journal of Applied Biosciences. 2010;**26**:1659-1663

[47] Latef AAHA, Jan S, Abd-Allah EF, Rashid B, John R, Ahmad P. Soybean under abiotic stress. In: Azooz MM, Ahmad P, editors. Plant-Environment Interaction: Responses and Approaches to Mitigate Stress. UK: John Wiley and Sons, Ltd; 2016

[48] Miransari M. Enhancing soybean response to biotic and abiotic stresses. In: Miransari M, editor. Abiotic and Biotic Stresses in Soybean Production, Soybean Production. Vol 1. UK: Academic Press Inc.; 2016. pp. 149-172

[49] Bhatnagar-Mathur P, Vadez V, Sharma KK. Transgenic approaches for abiotic stress tolerance in plants: Retrospect and prospects. Plant Cell Reports. 2008;**27**:411-424

[50] Condon AG, Richards RA, Rebetzke GL, Farguhar GD. Breeding for high water-use efficiency. Journal of Experimental Botany. 2004;**55**:2447-2460

[51] Mutava RN, Prince SJK, Syed NH, Song L, Valiyodun B, Chen W, Nguyen HT. Understanding abiotic stress tolerance mechanisms in soybean: A comparative evaluation of soybean response to drought and flooding stress. Plant Physiology and Biochemistry. 2015;**86**:109-120

[52] You J, Chan Z. ROS regulation during abiotic stress responses in crop plants. Frontiers in Plant Sciences. 2015;**6**(1092):1-15

[53] Mangena P. *Oryza* cystatin 1 based genetic transformation in soybean for drought tolerance. Masters' Dissertation. Sovenga, South Africa: University of Limpopo; 2015

[54] Khaine I, Woo SY. An overview of interrelationship between climate change and forests. Forest Science and Technology. 2015;**11**(1):11-18

[55] Kenrick P, Crane PR. The origin and early evolution of plants on land. Nature. 1997; **389**:33-39

[56] Xoconostle-Cazares B, Ramirez-Ortega FA, Flores-Elenes L, Ruiz-Medrano R. Drought tolerance in crop plants. American Journal of Plant Physiology. 2011;**5**(5):1-15

[57] Osakabe Y, Osakabe K, Shinozaki K, Tran LSP. Response of plants to water stress. Frontiers in Plant Science. 2014;**5**(86):1-8

[58] Gill SS, Tuteja N. Reactive oxygen species and antioxidant machinery in abiotic stress tolerance in crop plants. Plant Physiology and Biochemistry. 2010;**48**(12):909-930

[59] Hopkins WG. Introduction to Plant Physiology. 2nd ed. USA: John Wiley and Sons, Inc; 1999. pp. 189-214

[60] Simpson MG. Plant Systematics. USA: Elsevier Inc; 2010. pp. 535-539

[61] Zhang JZ, Creelman RA, Zhu JK. From laboratory to field. Using information from *Arabidopsis* to engineer salt, cold and drought tolerance in crops. Plant Physiology. 2004; **135**(2):615-621

[62] Montero-Tavera V, Ruiz-Medrano R, Xoconostle-Cazares B. Systematic nature of drought-tolerance in common bean. Plant Signaling & Behavior. 2008;**3**(9):663-666

[63] Abenavoli MR, Leone M, Sunseri F, Bacchi M, Sorgona A. Root phenotyping for drought tolerance in bean landraces from Calabria (Italy). Journal of Agronomy and Crop Science. 2015;**202**(1):1-12

[64] Nakashima K, Suenaga K. Review: Toward the genetic improvement of drought tolerance in crops. Japan International Research Quarterly. 2017;**51**(1):1-10

[65] Liu Z, Jin-Park B, Kanno A, Kameya T. The novel use of combination of sonication and vacuum infiltration in *Agrobacterium*-mediated transformation of kidney bean (*Phaseolus vulgaris* L.) with lea gene. Molecular Breeding. 2005;**16**:189-197

[66] Saijo Y, Hata S, Kyozula J, Shimamoto K, Izui K. Over-expression of a single Ca^{2+}-dependent protein kinase confers both cold and salt/ drought tolerance on rice plants. The Plant Journal. 2000;**23**(3):319-327

[67] Shou H, Bardallo P, Wang K. Expression of the *Nicotiana* protein kinase (NPK_1) enhanced drought tolerance in transgenic maize. Journal of Experimental Botany. 2004;**55**(399): 1013-1019

[68] Ku YS, Au-Yeung WK, Yung YL, Li MW, Wen CQ, Liu X, Lam HM. Drought stress and tolerance in soybean. In: Board JE, editor. A Comparative Survey of International Soybean Research: Genetics, Physiology, Agronomy and Nitrogen Relationships. Rijeka, Croatia: InTech Open; 2013. pp. 209-237

Chapter 3

Adaptation to Water Stress in Soybean: Morphology to Genetics

Tuanjie Zhao, Muqadas Aleem and
Ripa Akter Sharmin

Additional information is available at the end of the chapter

http://dx.doi.org/10.5772/intechopen.72229

Abstract

Soybean (*Glycine max* L.) is the most important legume and oilseed crop. As a leguminous crop, it plays an irreplaceable role towards the sustainable agricultural system with biological nitrogen fixation. However, its production can be dramatically decreased by the occurrence of water stress. Water stress including drought and flooding induces the morpho-physiological and biochemical changes at different growth stages, which negatively affects the adaptability and yield of soybean. Genetic diversity that ensures productivity in challenging environment exists within germplasm, their wild relatives and species that are adapted to the water stress. The discovery of gene mapping, QTLs associated with root traits, slow canopy wilting, nitrogen fixation and flooding tolerance have accomplished significant progress in breeding programs. Identification of drought-responsive genes and transcription factors such as *WRKY, DREBs, ERFs, ZIP, ZFP, MYB* and *NAC* are valuable to ameliorate the water stress in soybean. Understanding the genetic mechanism using transcriptomic and proteomic approaches would be the ultimate choice for mitigating the water stress. Integration of well-designed soybean breeding program coupled with omic techniques would pave the way for developing drought and flooding resilient soybean cultivars.

Keywords: soybean, drought, flooding, stress tolerance, quantitative trait locus, genomics, genetic diversity

1. Introduction

Soybean is an important leguminous crop in the world, providing an essential source of protein to human diet, feed for live-stock and as bio-diesel for industry [1, 2]. Soybean seeds consist of 40% protein, 20% oil, 35% carbohydrate and ~5% ash [3]. As compared to other oilseed crops, soybean collectively occupies around 6% of the world's land under cultivation [4].

Due to the rapid rise in the commercial value of soybean in an international market, the total area under soybean cultivation has been increasing from last three decades. Soybean is an important cash crop with a total production of over 313.05 million metric tons in 2015–2016 (USDA data). During this year, the USA has been the world's leading producer of soybean representing 35% of the world production, followed by Brazil with 31%, Argentina with 17%, China with 4%, India with 3%, Paraguay with 3% and Canada with 2% (USDA data).

Water stress including drought and flooding is considered as a major threat, limiting growth and yield of plants [5, 6]. Drought is caused by insufficient rainfall or irrigation which results in soil drying, whereas, in flooding, water exists in soil solution causing water logging and submergence. In response to drought and flooding stress, 40–60% yield losses have been reported in soybean [7, 8]. High temperature, low humidity in atmosphere and water deficiency are the main causes of drought [9, 10]. Drought stress affects germination rate and early seedling growth of the plant [11, 12]. Under water deficit conditions, a significant reduction in germination, hypocotyl length, root and shoot fresh and dry weight were observed whereas the root length is increased [13]. It also affects the carbon assimilation and phenology of the plant [10]. Prolonged drought stress at different growth stages has profound effect on soybean growth and yield [14].

To counteract the adverse effects of drought, the soybean plant adopts three mechanisms i.e. escape, tolerance, and avoidance [15]. In the escape mechanism, the plant completes its life cycle before the onset of drought. Normally, the plants complete their life cycle very quickly and produce few seeds. For instance, early planting of soybean helps to avoid drought, and is largely practiced in the USA—planting in March to April affords escape from water stress [16, 17]. Drought avoidance is performed by maintaining high water potential, grow deeper in soil, stomatal control of transpiration rate, and by reduction of water loss from tissues. The tolerance mechanism includes low tissue water potential, maintenance of turgor through osmotic adjustments [18, 19].

Flooding ranks second after drought, causing yield reduction in soybean [20, 21]. Flooding stress can be categorized as waterlogging or submergence. In waterlogging stress, root goes under water while shoots remains above ground, whereas, during submergence, plant is completely immersed in water saturated soil. As plants are aerobic, hypoxia (insufficient oxygen) or anoxia (complete absence of oxygen) causes losses in crop production. Soybean is more sensitive to flooding stress resulting in yield decline by reducing photosynthesis nitrogen fixation and biomass accumulation. Flooding stress can happen during any growing stage, especially in the seed germination and vegetative stages leads to substantial decrease of soybean grain yield [22] (**Table 1**). In addition, flooding stress hampers yield production during vegetative (17–43%) and reproductive stage (50–56%) [41].

For mitigating the negative impact of flooding stress, plants use a number of strategies for their survival, mainly escape and quiescence strategies [42, 43]. In escape strategy, morphological (aerenchyma development, shoot elongation and adventitious root formation) and anatomical alterations allow the plant to exchange gas between cells and atmosphere. The Quiescence strategy suppresses morphological changes to save energy and resources and retard plant growth. This strategy depends on anaerobic energy production [42, 44].

Growth stage	Experimental material	Indicator	Ref.
Under drought stress			
Germination	4 Bulgarian lines & one USA variety	Germination, shoot and root length, fresh and dry weight	[23]
Germination	L17, M9, Clark, M7, Hobbit and Williams	Root and shoot length, germination rate and percentage of germination	[24]
Second trifoliate leaves	Jindou 21 (C12), Mengjin 1 (W05) and Union (C08)	Gas exchange, water relation parameters, total chlorophyll, proline contents of leaves, root xylem pH, plant growth and root traits	[25]
Third trifoliate leaf (V3)	A5409RG, Jackson and Prima 2000	Root architecture, shoot parameters	[26]
Flowering and pod-filling stage	Habit, L17 and M17	Leaf relative water content, chemical osmolytes and chlorophyll content	[27]
V4, R1 and R3 growth stages.	Eight soybean cultivars	Highest number of node/plant, number of pod/main stem, pod/sub stem and pod/plant	[28]
Reproductive stage (R6–R7)	41 soybean accessions	increases in metaxylem number	[29, 30]
Adult	PI578477A,PI088444,PI458020	Yield, root architecture	[31]
Adult	BARI Soybean 5, BARI Soybean 6, Shohag and BD2331	relative performance (RP), tolerance (TOL), drought susceptibility index (DSI)	[32]
Under flooding stress			
Seedlings stage	Soybean	Secondary aerenchyma formation	[33]
Seedling stage	11 soybean genotypes	Primary/adventitious roots and root nodules, stem and leaf biomass	[34] [35]
Vegetative and flowering stage	Taekwang and Asoaogari	Root morphological traits, adventitious roots and Photosynthesis	[36]
Cotyledon-stage seedlings	92 Soybean Lines	Root architecture	[37]
Flowering stage	Cultivars Fundacep 53 RR and BRS Macota	Fermentative metabolism and carbohydrate contents in roots and nodules	[38]
Flowering stage	Five soybean cultivars	Nodule number, nodule dry weight, chlorophyll content, carbon exchange rate, dry matter accumulation and nitrogen content	[39]
Seedling stage	162 soybean accessions	Root development	[40]

Table 1. A list of drought- and flooding-related parameters at different growth stages of soybean.

Understanding the genetic base for water stress tolerance in diverse soybean is a fundamental issue that contributes for the genetic improvement. This chapter will present the research progress about the situation of soybean tolerance to water stress at germination, seedling and adult plant stages. It also includes the current knowledge about QTL mapping, gene discovery and 'omic' technologies relevant to drought and flooding tolerance that will be helpful to understand drought and flooding-tolerance mechanisms in soybean.

2. Genetic diversity of water stress tolerance in soybean

2.1. Different response of soybean to water stress

2.1.1. Morphological performance

Drought induces morphological changes in plants, enabling them to sense and rapidly adapt to the stress. Root-related traits are crucial in maintaining crop yield in soybean [45]. Drought alters the root system architecture (root depth, root angle and root branching density) [27]. For instance, root architecture was characterized in field under normal and water deficit conditions using three soybean cultivars (Jackson, Prima 2000 and A5409RG). As a result, Prima 2000 (drought-tolerant cultivar) has an intermediate root phenotype with a root angle of 40–60°, while a shallow root phenotype along with root angle of <40° has been observed in drought-sensitive cultivar A5409RG [27].

Depth of rooting system influenced by the elongation of taproot also plays an important role for plant survival under water deficit [27, 46]. An increase in number of root tips, root length, root surface area and root volume was observed under water limited conditions. Several studies have proposed that roots having large xylem number, diameters, lateral root systems with more root hairs are indicators of drought tolerance [31, 47, 48]. Jackson is considered as drought escaping cultivar with long and deep roots into the soil permitting better water uptake compared with drought-sensitive cultivars [27, 49]. Under water-limited conditions, Plant Introduction (PI) 578477A and 088444 exhibited higher yield due to higher lateral root number in clay soil [50]. It was reported that deeper region of soil has high root density under seasonal drought as compared to dry surface of soil [51]. In addition, total root length/ plant weight, dry root weight/plant weight and root volume/plant weight were positively correlated with drought tolerance [52]. Therefore, studying the relationship between root traits and drought is helpful to develop drought-resistant cultivar.

Root-to-shoot ratio is also a good indicator to allocate the resources between different plant components. The water-limited environment increases the root-to-shoot ratio. For example, in soybean, root-to-shoot ratio increased by 13% indicates the flow of biomass towards roots [53]. The drought-tolerant soybean genotype (C12) showed a higher root-to-shoot ratio than the susceptible genotype (C08) under restricted soil water with application of exogenous ABA. To cope with drought stress, leaf morphology also plays an important role. Under water-limited conditions, plants reduce their leaf area by closing stomata. Due to water scarcity, reduction in soybean plant leaf area has been reported [54]. In contrast, drought-tolerant soybean cultivar exhibited a greater leaf area rather than less-tolerant cultivar under hydric stress condition [55].

Aerenchyma formation is a major indicator that facilitates gas exchange between aerial and submerged plant parts (shoots and/or roots) to avoid flooding stress [56, 57]. Flooding stress induces two kinds of aerenchyma i.e. primary (cortical) [58] and secondary (white and spongy tissues) [33]. A number of aquatic plants develop cortical aerenchymatous tissue by cell disintegration (lysigenous aerenchyma) and cell separation (schizogenous aerenchyma) [59]. In rice, barley, maize and wheat, lysigenous aerenchyma is induced by flooding [60, 61]. In some species, especially in soybean, secondary aerenchyma having a spongy parenchyma cell layer develops through cell division of phellogen [44, 62]. Secondary aerenchyma is morphologically and anatomically different from cortical aerenchyma (lysigenous and schizogenous aerenchyma) [33]. Waterlogging stimulated the formation of aerenchyma and adventitious roots in soybean plants facilitating transport of oxygen from shoot to root [62–64]. Under waterlogging condition, adventitious roots are formed in several flooded plants including soybean [61, 62, 65]. However, adventitious roots are absent in soybean seedlings under complete submergence [66]. Under flooding conditions, secondary aerenchyma consisting of white and spongy tissues develops within a few weeks in stems, roots and root nodules of soybean [33]. Aerenchyma formations initiated by ethylene, Ca^{2+}, and ROS signalling through a programmed cell death process are involved in aerenchyma development [60, 67].

Rapid shoot elongation is another escape mechanism for adaptation in waterlogging stress [68]. It has been reported that lower stem of soybean having hypertrophic lenticels helps oxygen entry into the aerenchyma [64]. Flooding also causes a significant reduction in leaf number, leaf area, canopy height and dry weight at maturity in soybean crops.

2.1.2. Physiological and biochemical response under drought stress

Stress-responsive mechanisms have been studied at the physiological and biochemical level in soybean under drought and flooding stress. To optimize the use of water under water deficit conditions, stomatal control is considered as major physiological indicator. For instance, in soybean, stomatal conductance decreased by 42% in drought-stressed leaves rather than normal leaves [69]. Owing to dehydration, MG/BR46 (drought tolerant soybean variety) showed faster decline in stomatal conductance as compared to BR16 (drought-susceptible variety) (65 versus 50% reduction) [55]. In same study, prolonged drought stress (45 days) exhibited no profound impact on stomatal conductance of BR16 while it had reached 79% in the MG/BR46. Several studies have provided strong evidence that drought-tolerant soybean genotypes (C12 and W05) exhibited a higher reduction in stomatal conductance rather than the susceptible one (C08) [25]. In soybean, ABA is involved in the reduction of stomatal conductance and photosynthesis. For instance, after imposition of exogenous application of ABA under soil drying, leaf stomatal conductance of soybean tolerant genotype C12 declined than the susceptible one (C08).

Maintenance of cell turgidity and water-use efficiency are important indicators to cope with drought stress [26]. Soybean introduction line PI 416937 is an excellent example of drought tolerance by limiting transpiration rate and maintaining a lower osmotic potential. An increase in WUE was observed in drought-tolerant genotype (C12) by regulating stomatal closure during the entire period of water deficiency [25, 52].The maintenance of cell turgidity under water-limited conditions may be achieved by adjusting the osmotic potential in response to the accumulation of proline, sucrose, soluble carbohydrates, glycine betaine and other solutes [70]. The accumulation of solutes under water deficit condition is known as osmotic adjustment. Some authors have reported higher proline content in drought-tolerant crop species such as bean [71]. In soybean, water stress exhibited significant increase in proline contents in drought tolerance as well as susceptible genotype, but tolerant genotypes recovered to pre-stress levels more quickly after rehydration [25].

The production of ROS, such as superoxide radical (O_2^-), hydroxyl radical ($OH^\cdot$) and hydrogen peroxide (H_2O_2), is one of the biochemical responses causing damage to DNA, proteins and lipids [72] under drought stress. The toxicity of ROS may be limited by antioxidant enzymatic (superoxide dismutase, catalase, and glutathione peroxidase) and non-enzymatic scavengers [73, 74]. For instance, drought stress increased activities of some antioxidant enzymes (catalase, glutathione reductase and superoxide dismutase) in soybean varieties which were positively correlated to seed yield [75].

Under flooding stress, plant undergoes different physiological and biochemical adaptations. For instance, in soybean, a significant reduction in photosynthetic activity and stomatal conductance was observed in Essex and Forrest within 48 h of flooding at vegetative and reproductive growth stages. Waterlogging also decreases biological nitrogen fixation, as nodules need adequate oxygen to maintain nitrogenase activity for aerobic respiration and contributing adenosine triphosphate [41]. As a consequence of flooding stress, a reduction in root hydraulic conductivity has also been reported [76]. Several studies have provided the correlation between stomatal conductance and carbon fixation. In flooded plants, photosynthetic activities were reduced by restricting CO_2 due to stomatal closure [77, 78]. Furthermore, due to the higher concentration of CO_2 assimilation in flooded soil, biomass and soybean root elongation eventually repressed [79].

Tamang et al. [66] reported that submergence stimulates starch degradation, soluble carbohydrates and ATP in cotyledons and hypocotyls of soybean seedlings. Extensive submergence degrades the chlorophyll contents in aerial parts of several terrestrial plants [80, 81]. However, under submergence, abundance of chlorophyll *a* and *b* remained nearly constant in soybean [66]. The decrease in photosynthetic activity with long-term flooding may be triggered by the reduction in chlorophyll, transpiration and ribulose-1,5-biphosphate (RuBP) carboxylase activity. These combined effects against flooding declined the crop growth, net assimilation and leaf expansion of plants. Blocking of hypertrophic lenticels at the base of stem restricted O_2 transport into the roots resulting in reduction of plant growth under hypoxic conditions [82]. Flooding stress causes higher production of ROS resulting in oxidative damage to proteins related to photosynthetic apparatus [83]. As a result, the scavenging activity is overpassed under flooding stress.

2.2. Parameters for measuring the tolerance degree of water stress

2.2.1. Parameters related to seed tolerance

Seeds need a suitable condition to have a good germination. The germination rate and percentage of different cultivars were affected by levels of drought stress. In soybean, drought stress simulated by polyethylene glycol PEG-6000 significantly reduced seed germination percentage (**Table 1**). An increase in the PEG concentration reduced root growth by two to three times for different genotypes. Seed weight and seed size, and seed weight distribution are key indicators to evaluate the genotypic response to drought stress [84, 85]. A positive correlation between 100-seed weight per plant and seed yield were reported in soybean under water limited conditions. For instance, Habit (soybean drought-tolerant cultivar) exhibited higher 100-seed weight and seed yield under drought stress [29, 86].Water deficit conditions lead to a significant reduction in seed weight and seed size. It also had little effect on seed shape as shrunken and wrinkled, and hard seeds were produced in soybean [84, 85, 87]. Same study pointed out 30–40% reduction in proportion of seed having diameter > 4.8 mm. In contrast, the ratio of seeds of diameter < 3.2 mm was increased by 3–15% [85].

Germination is a complex process that consists of several metabolic events. Numerous studies reported that negative correlation exists between germination percentage and flooding stress [88, 89]. Seeds are usually germinated under optimum conditions within 1 or 2 days. But, seed germination is delayed due to the quick absorption of water, collapse of seed structure, and outflow of internal seed contents under flooding stress. When seeds were flooded for 3 days after imbibition, germination percentage was drastically dropped out and seed injury was observed [90]. Flooding causes mechanical damage on the soybean seeds and prohibits germination. Seed coat and seed weight are fundamental factors to evaluate a positive effect on seed flooding tolerance. For example, germination rate (GR) and normal seedling rate (NS) was higher in pigmented varieties as compared to yellow varieties of soybean (**Table 1**). These parameters (GR and NS) were negatively correlated with seed weight (SW) in the combined population [91]. Therefore, pigmented seed coat and small seed weight could be key parameters in response to seed-flooding tolerance.

2.2.2. Parameters related to vegetative tissues

Root length, shoot length and leaf area are considered as major determinants to evaluate drought response during vegetative stage. A positive relationship exists between root traits and resistance to drought [52, 92]. At seedling stage, drought stress affects leaf expansion rate, leaf water potential, relative water content of leaves (%RWC) and relative growth. The degradation of chlorophyll contents of soybean leaves was correlated with the different levels of drought stress [75]. Water deficit stress also decreased the number of nodes and intermodal length while the reduction in inter-nodal length depends upon the duration of drought stress. For example, drought stress showed no profound impact on number of internodes in drought tolerant soybean cultivar (C12), whereas drought-susceptible cultivar (C08) showed higher number of internode [93].

Essential traits, root length and shoot length are also important indicators in response to flooding stress. The insufficient allocation of water, minerals, nutrients, and hormones led to root and shoot damage [94]. The first symptom usually appears in soybean is wilting of leaves in response to flooding. Soybean shoot growth under flooded conditions is significantly decreased due to inability of the root system regarding water transport, hormones, nutrients and assimilates [95, 96]. Flooding tolerance in soybean is strongly correlated to root surface area, root length and dry weight [97]. It has been reported that root tips are extremely sensitive to flooding in soybean and pea seedlings [98–100]. Under complete submergence, soybean root growth is absolutely repressed due to the death of root tips.

2.2.3. Parameters related to adult plants

In soybean, pod number per plant, seed number per pod and 100-seed weight are major determinants of yield under water stress [101], and these yield components are the important sink for assimilates at reproductive stages [102]. Drought stress especially during flowering (R1) and pod-filling stages reduces soybean yield [30] (**Table 1**). Under water deficit conditions, an increase in rate of abortion has been reported during early pod-filling stage in soybean [54, 103]. Soybean yield is also affected by the occurrence of drought stress during seed filling (R6) period [93]. Water stress at flowering stage decreased the pod number and seed number resulting in yield loss [104]. Kobraei et al. [29] conducted experiment on eight soybean cultivars to asses yield under normal and drought conditions. This study pointed out that drought reduced the yield components resulting in yield loss. In addition, more yield loss was observed during R1 stage as compared to R6 stage [104].

One of the major traits conferring tolerance to waterlogging is yield and production of good quality seeds [105]. A significant decline in pod number, pods per node, branch number, and seed size was observed following 7 days of flooding at different vegetative and regenerative development stages [106]. Sullivan et al. [107] confirmed reduction in pod number and plant height at early vegetative growth stages. Soybean crops flooded with excessive water at early flowering stage showed severe chlorosis and stunting growth [108]. Schöffel et al. [109] showed a decreased number of pods per plant at the reproductive stage (R4) in pot trails. A field experiment was conducted in flooded soil and obtained yield reduction from 20–39% in the different soybean cultivars when subjected during the R5 stage. During flooding, a significant reduction in soybean yield was observed at R5 stage as compared to the R2 stage [110].

2.3. Genetic variation of tolerance to water stress

2.3.1. Cultivated soybean

Considerable genetic variation in seed yield was observed in soybean genotypes under drought stress. A total of 50 soybean genotypes were screened under rain-fed condition in Bangladesh. Among them, genotypes BARI Soybean 5, BARI Soybean 6, Shohag and BD2331 were identified as drought-tolerant genotypes [32]. In another study, response of eight cultivars of soybean (Clark, Hobbit, Pershing, Williams, Hood, DPX, M7 and M9) was investigated in Iran. Williams cultivar was predicted as drought-tolerant, having highest number of nodes and pods/plant in normal and water deficit conditions [29]. Genetically and geographically, diverse soybean germplasm lines i.e. from Korea (PI085355, PI339984, PI407778A, PI407973A, PI423841, PI424460, PI424608A, PI603170, PI458020), China (PI088444, PI567398, PI567561, PI594410, PI578477A), Japan (PI243548, PI417092, PI507066) were screened to examine root response under water deficit condition in clay and sandy soil. Plant Introduction PI578477A, PI088444 (high lateral root number in clay soil) and PI458020 (thick lateral roots in sandy soil) were found to have higher yield under water-limited conditions [50]. Brazilian cultivars BR-4 and Ocepar 4 were considered as drought-tolerant [111]. Several cultivated germplasm lines (*Glycine max*) including Williams, Jackson, Prima 2000, Jindou 21(C12), PI416937, PI 427136, PI 408105A, PI 471938, PI 424088, PI 081041, N04-9646, DT51 and R02-1325 have promising performance under water deficit conditions and can be used in breeding program [25, 27, 112, 113].

Genetic variation in soybean germplasm was observed in response to flooding tolerance to overcome yield loss. Elite lines conserve genomic regions that can inhibit extensive yield losses during flooding stress. An experiment was conducted to determine genetic variations using 21 soybean varieties for flooding tolerance in both screen-house and field tests. Three soybean germplasm, Nam Vang from Cambodia, VND2 from China and ATF15-1 from Australia were identified as most flood-tolerant varieties which survived better, grew taller, produced more pods/plants and heavier seed weight as compared to sensitive varieties [114]. A total of 192 soybean germplasm lines were screened for flooding tolerance at seedling stage. Among them, Jangbaegkong, Danbaegkong, Sowonkongkong, Socheong2 and Suwon269 were identified as donor line for flooding tolerance, whereas Shillog, T201, T181, NTS1116 and HP-963 exposed flooding sensitivity [115]. Several cultivated germplasm lines (*Glycine max*) including PI 408105A, PI 561271, PI 567343, PI 407184, PI603910C, PI 567394B, PI 567651, Archer and Misuzudaiz have been identified as a source of potential source for flooding tolerance [112].

2.3.2. *Wild soybean*

Wild soybean (*Glycine soja*), is a valuable genetic resource for the tolerance to water stress by reintroducing alleles. Wild soybean PI 483463 (*G. soja*) had favourable donor alleles for root angle, while PI 468917 predicted to contribute to slow wilting. Hence, it can be used for development of drought-resistant soybean cultivars [112, 116]. In another study, the wild parent, PI 407162 had favourable alleles for fibrous roots, thus enhancing the soybean ability to survive under drought stress. These studies suggested that it is possible to enhance genetic variation in cultivated soybean by introducing alleles from wild soybeans [117]. For flooding, different wild soybean accessions, PI 467162, PI 479751, PI 407229, PI 597459C, PI 424082, PI 378699A, PI 424107A, PI 366124, PI 378699A were identified, which showed tremendous waterlogging tolerance than *G. max* [112]. Therefore, wild populations can offer useful in breeding program for improving drought and flooding resistance of soybean.

3. Genetic regulation mechanisms for tolerance to water stress

3.1. Drought tolerance

3.1.1. *Genetic and QTL structure of morpho-physiological performance*

The application of QTL helps in identification of chromosomal regions, detecting phenotypic variation associated with drought-resistance traits and to determine the desirable alleles at these QLs for marker-assisted breeding. Progress towards the identification of drought-related QTLs is needed [118], only a few QTLs have been reported for drought (**Table 2**). Du et al. [128] identified 19 QTLs associated with seed yield under normal and water-limited conditions and 10 QTLs associated with drought susceptibility index (DSI) in soybean. To develop drought-tolerant varieties, the role of secondary traits associated with yield stability has been accelerated. In crops, under water deficit condition, several secondary traits i.e. early seedling vigor [129], canopy wilting [119, 130], root system architecture (RSA) [117, 131, 132], canopy temperature depression [133], carbon isotope discrimination [134, 135], alterations in photosynthesis [136, 137], and nitrogen fixation [138–141] have been reported.

In soybean, RSAs, slow canopy wilting and biological nitrogen fixation are promising secondary traits under drought [112]. Under water deficit conditions, a simulation analysis model depicted that slow wilting can improve soybean yield >75% while nitrogen fixation up to 85% [142]. In soybean, less information is available on QTL mapping of drought-associated traits and yield [128, 143], fibrous roots [144] and water-use efficiency (WUE) [123, 125, 126] under water-limited conditions. Several studies have been conducted on QTL mapping for RSA traits in major cereals crops with little information in leguminous crops, especially soybean [145–147]. Five QTLs were identified on chromosomes 1, 3, 4, 8, and 20 related with fibrous rooting systems in RIL population of soybean derived from a cross between Benning (low fibrous root) and PI 416937 (extensive fibrous root) [144]. These QTLs were detected by using 240 F6 derived recombinant inbred lines (RILs) under rain-fed conditions for 2 years (2001 and 2009). The parent PI 416937 (extensive fibrous root system) contributed favourable alleles for four QTLs, while one QTL had donor alleles from Benning. Moreover, a total of four QTLs related with root surface area and distribution (based on root length and thickness) were identified in an inter-specific mapping population (*Glycine max* × *Glycine soja*). Two QTLs on Chr 6 had favourable donor alleles from the wild parent, PI 407162 (*G. soja*) with R2 value of >10%. As a result, plants enhanced their ability to form fibrous roots. Manavalan et al. [148] identified one QTL cluster associated with root length and lateral root number in 251 BC2F5 backcross inbred lines through linkage mapping with favourable alleles from Dunbar (**Table 2**).

Slow canopy wilting is a key factor to screen soybean germplasm under water-limited conditions [121]. A total of 13 QTLs associated with slow wilting were detected using five bi-parental populations under water-limited conditions, with phenotypic variation (R2 0.04–0.29). Eleven out of 13 QTLs had favourable alleles from PI 416937 and Jackson [119–121]. The major QTL associated with slow wilting was mapped on LG K with 17% phenotypic variation [122]. To validate QTL data from different mapping population on same linkage map, 'Meta-QTL analysis' has been proposed [149, 150]. In soybean, Meta-QTL analysis was used to refine the confidence interval of eight QTLs using mapping results from five bi-parental population However, these QTLs are complex, unstable and quantitative nature, so breeders find difficulties to utilize them [151]. Considering this problem, confirmation of QTL should be performed by using more advanced progeny or near isogenic lines (BC_nF_2).

Studies on QTL mapping associated with biological-nitrogen fixation are very few in plants including soybean. Three QTLs for nodule number (LGs B1, E) were identified using the composite interval mapping and explained 13% phenotypic variation [152]. Two QTLs for shoot ureide were detected on Chrs. 9 and 19, and two QTLs associated with shoot nitrogen concentration were mapped on Chrs. 13 and 17 under water stress. These QTLs explained phenotypic variation ranging from 0.11 to 0.31 (**Table 2**) [127]. Jackson contributed favourable alleles for shoot ureide concentration on Gm 19 and Gm 13 while other two on Gm 09 and Gm17 have favourable alleles from KS4895. Under well-watered conditions, a number of QTLs associated with shoot ureide and nitrogen concentrations were reported. However, not a single QTL was detected under both conditions (stress and control) illustrating that soybean shows diverse mechanisms for regulation of N_2-fixation under well-watered and drought conditions [127].

Trait	QTL	Chro.	Marker	R^2	Population	Ref.
Canopy wilting	*Gm02-1*	2	ss107913715	0.06–0.12	KJ, BP	[119]
	Gm02-2	2	ss107912946/satt296	0.06–0.18	AP	[119, 120]
	Gm02-3	2	Satt296	0.06–0.19	BP, AP	[119]
	qSW-Gm04	4	Satt646	0.09	BP	[120]
	Gm05	5	ss107913925/satt276	0.04–0.16	KJ	[119, 120]
	Gm08	8	Satt177	0.05–0.15	KJ, KN	[119, 121]
Leaf wilting	*Gm09*	9	Sat044	0.17	Jackson ×KS4895	[122]
Canopy wilting	*Gm11*	11	ss107913507	0.14–0.39	KJ, KP, AP	[119]
	qSW-Gm12	12	Satt302	0.27	BP	[120]
	Gm13	13	Satt362	0.16	KJ	[121]
	Gm14	14	ss107913401	0.08–0.12	KJ,AP	[119, 121]
	qSW-Gm17/ Gm17–1	17	ss107929993	0.06–0.22	KJ,AP, BP	[119–121]
	Gm17-2	17	ss107913610	0.09–0.10	KJ, KP	[119]
	qSW-Gm19	19	ss107924069	0.11–0.29	KJ, KP, BP	[119]
Yield	*Gm06*	6	Satt205-satt489	0.7	Minsoy ×Noir 1	[123]
Yield and wilting	*Gm13*	13	Sat_375	–	Hutcheson × PI471938,	[124]
	Gm13-1	13	Sat_074	–		
	Gm17	17	Satt226	–		
Water use efficiency	*Gm19*	19	A489H	0.14	S-100 × Tokyo	[125]
	–	–	A063-1	0.8		
	Gm18	18	B031-1	8.5	Young ×PI416937	[126]
	Gm12	12	A089-1	8.7		
	Gm16	16	cr497-1	13.2		
	Gm16	16	K375-1	7.5		
	Gm4	4	A063-1	5		
Nitrogen fixation (shoot ureide)	*Gm09*	9	BARC-060299-16,598	0.16	KS4895 × Jackson	[127]
	Gm19	19	Satt561	0.18		
	Gm13	13	BARC-014657-01608	0.24		
	Gm17	17	BARC-057467-14,765	0.12		

KJ = KS4895 × Jackson; BP = Benning × PI 416937; AP = A5959 × PI 416937; KP = KS4895 × PI 424140; KN = Kefeng1 × Nannong1138-2.

Table 2. A list of reported QTLs in soybean associated with drought tolerance.

3.1.2. Identification of important genes for drought tolerance

Drought stress-responsive genes are categorized as effectors and regulatory genes [153]. Effectors include gene encoding protein such as LEA proteins, osmolyte biosynthesis (osmotin), aquaporins, chaperons, antioxidants and enzymes involved in different metabolic pathway. Regulatory genes encoding product such as receptors, calmodulin-binding proteins, kinases, phosphatases and transcription factors are involved in signal transduction and gene expression [153]. A number of plant TFs such as ethylene-responsive factor, WRKY, MYB, basic leucine zipper domain (bZIP) and NAC are involved in ABA signalling under drought stress, while dehydration responsible element binding (DREB) protein, are involved in ABA-independent pathway [154–156]. Major families of TF genes expressed in response to drought stress in plants are summarized in **Table 3**.

In the soybean genome, 5035 TFs models were identified based on in-silico annotation [170]. Among all TFs, the WRKY transcription factor is the largest family in plants. A total of 233 WRKY members have been identified in soybean (http://planttfdb.cbi.pku.edu.cn/family.php?fam=WRKY) [171]. Identification of two WRKY genes (GmWRKY21 and GmWRKY54) and their role in enhancing tolerance to drought, salt and cold has been studied in *Arabidopsis* [156]. Moreover, the involvement of GmWRKY27 has been characterized under drought and salt stress. Overexpression of GmWRKY27 RNAi and GmWRKY27 in soybeans results in increased tolerance and hypersensitivity to drought and salt stress, respectively. In the same study, the association of GmWRKY27 with GmMYB174 was observed, which binds to neighbouring cis-elements

Gene family	Gene	Studied plant	Ref.
R2R3-MYB transcription factor	GmMYB84	Soybean	[157]
	GmMYBJ1	Arabidopsis	[158]
bZIP transcription factor	GmFDL19	Soybean	[159]
	GmbZIP1	Arabidopsis	[160]
DREB transcription factor	GmDREB2	Tobacco	[161]
AP2/ERF transcription factor	GmDREB2A;2	Soybean	[162]
AP2/ERF transcription factor	GmERF3	Tobacco	[163]
AP2/ERF transcription factor	GmERF4	Tobacco	[164]
WRKY family	GmWRKY54	Arabidopsis	[156]
WRKY family	GsWRKY20	Arabidopsis	[165]
NAC family	GmNAC20	Soybean	[166]
Homeodomainleucine zipper (HD-Zip) proteins	Multiple HD-Zip genes	Soybean	[167]
C_2H_2-type Zinc finger protein	GmZFP3	Arabidopsis	[168]
Trihelix transcription factors	GmGT-2B b	Arabidopsis	[169]
	GmGT-2A	Arabidopsis	

Table 3. Major families of TF genes expressed in response to drought stress in plants.

in GmNAC29 promoter and suppressed gene expression of GmNAC29 led to increased tolerance to abiotic stress [172]. In soybean, novel candidates of WRKY genes were detected, which provided the unique function of WRKY transcription factors under water deficit conditions [173].

Another gene family, Homeodomain-leucine zipper (HD-Zip) comprised of 140 HD-Zip genes (http://planttfdb.cbi.pku.edu.cn/family.php?fam=HD-ZIP) were detected under drought and salt stress. Out of 140, 59 are coding genes while 20 paralogous genes exhibited differential expression under drought and saline environment [174]. In soybean, overexpression of GmDREB3 also enhances tolerance drought tolerance in response to accumulation of proline [175].

3.2. Flooding tolerance

3.2.1. QTL mapping

In recent years, the advent of molecular marker technologies has opened up new opportunities for QTL analyses, fine mapping and cloning of genes for water stress tolerance. The genetic basis of drought and flooding tolerance has been studied by evaluating different component traits in drought and flood-tolerant soybean. Both drought and flooding tolerance are quantitatively inherited and controlled by several genetic loci. Consequently, a large number of QTLs related to flooding tolerance are summarized in **Table 4**.

The analysis of quantitative trait loci (QTLs) for water-logging tolerance in soybean is usually challenging. However, several studies have been done on QTLs associated to flooding tolerance, focused on injury score and tolerance index in soybean [91, 176–179, 182]. For instance, a single QTL located on Chr. 18 (Sat_064) was identified using 208 lines of two recombinant inbred (RI) populations, for soybean growth and grain yields under water-logging conditions [176].

Trait	QTL	Chro.	Marker	Population	Ref.
Grain yield	*Gm18*	18	Sat_064	Archer × Minsoy, Archer × Noir I	[176]
Injury score, tolerance index	*Gm5, Gm13*	5, 13	Satt385, Satt269	A5403 × Archer, P9641 × Archer	[177]
Flooding tolerance	*ft1*	6	Satt100	Misuzudaizu × Gong 503	[178]
Seed germination	*Sft1, Sft2*	12, 8	Sat_175, Satt 187	Peking × Tamahomare	[91]
	Sft3, Sft4	4, 2	Satt 338, Sat_279		
Flooding toleranceand/or resistance to *P. sojae*	*FTS-13*	13	Sct_033, BARC-024569-4982	PI 408105A × S99-2281	[179]
	FTS-11	11	BARC-016279-02316		
Joint waterlogging tolerance index	*Wt1,wt2*	19	Satt229-Satt527 Satt527-Sat_286	Su88-M21 × Xinyixiaoheidou	[180]
Root length development/ Root surface area	*Qhti-12-1*	12	Satt052-Satt302	Iyodaizu × Tachinagaha	[181]

Table 4. A summary of QTL mapping studies for flood tolerance traits in soybean.

The results indicated that the Sat_064 QTL is unique in response to flooding. The Sat_064 QTL was further confirmed in a southern cultivar Archer using near-isogenic lines (NILs) [183]. In addition, two flooding-tolerance QTLs on Chr. 5 (Satt385) and Chr.13 (Satt269) were identified associated with water-logging tolerance through partial linkage mapping and bulk-segregation analysis using two populations [177]. Seven loci were detected associated with yield in response to flooding in a mapping population between Misuzudaizu and Moshidou Gong 503. Among them, only a large and stable QTL, *ft1* tightly linked with flowering was reproducible with high LOD score in 2 years, 2012 and 2013 (15.41 and 7.57) [178].

In another experiment, four QTLs, *Sft1, Sft2, Sft3 and Sft4* associated with seed-flooding tolerance, during geminating stage, were detected using population derived from cross between a tolerant 'Peking' (black seed coat) × susceptible cultivar 'Tamahomare' (yellow seed coat). Among these QTLs, *Sft1* located on Chr.12 had great effect on germination rate, whereas *sft2* mapped on Chr. 8 had contribution in seed coat pigmentation [91]. Two QTLs, *FTS-11* and *FTS-13* were mapped on Chr. 11 and Chr.13, respectively, using F_7 recombinant inbred lines (RILs) at an early reproductive stage. These QTLs were also related with flooding yield index and flooding injury score. The major QTL *FTS-13*, with phenotypic variation 18.3% was detected in multiple locations and years [179]. Recently, QTLs for root surface area development (RSAD) and root length development (RLD) on Chr. 12 (between markers Satt052 and Satt302) were identified in relation to hypoxia tolerance using F8:9 RILs derived from a cross between Iyodaizu and Tachinagaha in soybean. For the validation of these major and stable QTLs, NILs with the QTL region were developed derived from Iyodaizu [181].

3.2.2. *Transcriptome analysis of soybean under water stress*

Transcript abundance analysis is vital functional genomics tools to examine flooding responsive mechanisms and identify genes responsible for flooding tolerance. Recently, genome-wide changes associated with gene-expression are investigated through microarray chip analysis, RNA-seq approach and high-coverage gene expression profiling analysis for better understanding the transcriptional response in relation to flooding stress in soybean (**Table 5**). Transcripts were examined in the root tip, including the hypocotyl of soybean, using high-coverage gene expression profiling analysis; 5831 out of 29,388 were significantly altered under water stress. Genes relevant to ethylene biosynthesis, alcoholic fermentation and cell wall relaxation are promptly up-regulated in response to flooding. Defence-related genes, haemoglobin, and Kunitz trypsin protease inhibitor and acid phosphatase are responsible for flooding [184].

In another study, soybean microarray chip-based transcriptomics technique was used to comprehend the molecular response under flooding. In soybean roots including hypocotyl, more than 6000 flooding-responsive genes were identified. The results revealed that genes associated with glycolysis, photosynthesis, amino acid synthesis (Ser-Gly-Cys group), transcriptional regulation of transcription, degradation of ubiquitin-mediated protein, and cell death were expressively up-regulated, whereas genes relevant to cell organization, secondary metabolism, cell wall synthesis, transport of metabolite and chromatin structure were considerably down-regulated. Furthermore, up-regulation of flooding-responsive genes encoding small proteins plays key roles in acclimation to flooding [185]. It has been reported that a total of 2724 and

Stress	Tissues	Platform	DEG*/proteins characterized	Ref
Flooding	Root and hypocotyl	High coverage expression profiling	97 genes and 34 proteins	[184]
Flooding	Roots including hypocotyl	Soybean microarray chip	More than 6000 genes	[185]
Drought & flooding	Leaf tissue	Illumina Genome Analyzer (San Die go, CA) platform	2724 genes for drought and 3498 genes for flooding, 289 Transcription Factors	[186]
Flooding stress	Root tips, root with hypocotyl and cotyledons	RNA sequencing-based transcriptomic analysis	31 genes	[187]
Drought & flooding	Leaf, hypocotyl, and root	Gel-free/label-free proteomic technique	17 proteins	[188]
Drought & flooding	Roots	Gel-free proteomic technique	97 proteins in response to flooding and 48 proteins for drought	[189]
Drought & flooding	Root tip	Gel-free/label-free proteomic analysis	Three S-adenosylmethionine synthetases (SAMs) proteins	[190]
Flooding	Root and cotyledon	Nano spray LTQ XL Orbitrap mass spectrometry (MS)	146 proteins	[191]
Flooding & drought	Roots	Gel-free proteomic technique	97 proteins to flooding, 48 for drought	[189]

*Differentially Expressed Gene.

Table 5. Soybean transcriptome and proteome studies under flooding and drought stress.

3498 genes were differentially expressed in response to drought and flooding stress, respectively, which contain 289 TFs demonstrating ethylene response factors (ERFs), basic helix-loop helix (bHLH), WRKY amino acid motif (WRKY), myeloblastosis (MYB) and no apical meristem (NAC) are involved in stress tolerance mechanism [186].

RNA-seq based transcriptomic analysis resulted in detection of 729 and 255 genes in the flooding-tolerant line and ABA-treated soybean, respectively, which were significantly changed under stress condition. Transcript profiles also revealed that a total of 31 genes included 12 genes involved in the regulation of RNA and protein metabolism were commonly altered between the flooding-tolerant line and ABA-treated soybean under flooding stress [187]. On the basis of the above findings, it can be concluded that transcript profiles can be helpful as an adaptive mechanism for soybean survival under water stress.

3.2.3. Proteomics techniques for identification of water stress-responsive mechanisms

Different proteomics techniques i.e. mass spectroscopy (MS)-based (for identification of a number of environmental stress-responsive proteins), two-dimensional (2D) gel-based (for visual illustration of the proteins) and SDS gel or gel free-based (for detection of the largest number of proteins) are extensively used under water stress (**Table 5**). The available genomic information in soybean genome database helps to identify water stress-responsive mechanism. Distinct changes in the soybean proteome during water stress lead to different defence mechanisms. Several studies evidently revealed that some proteins regulating sucrose accumulation, glucose degradation, cell wall relaxing, signal transduction and alcohol fermentation were altered under flooding stress [192, 193]. Flooding stress reduced the differential regulation of proteins involved in maintaining the structure of cell and protein folding [99]. Moreover, the application of exogenous calcium on flooded soybeans up-regulated the lipid metabolism, signalling-related proteins, glycolysis-related proteins and fermentation in roots [189]. A reduction in calcium oxalate crystals was found in cotyledon under flooding [188].

Wang et al. identified three *S*-adenosylmethionine synthetases (SAMs) proteins using gel-free proteomic analysis under water stress in soybean. The SAMs action declined at early-stage flooding but increased in hypocotyls and roots under water deficit. The results recommended that SAMs were involved in response to water stress and it might affect ethylene biosynthesis in soybean. The action of SAMs was different in hypocotyls, root tips and roots under water stress. The down-regulation of *SAMs 1* and *SAMs 2* were observed in roots under drought and flooding. Moreover, up-regulation of ACC synthase was examined under drought, whereas the expression was down-regulated in root tips under flooding. However, ACC oxidase was increased under both stresses. These findings indicate that SAMs have key role in ethylene biosynthesis in soybean [194]. A quantitative proteomics study has been conducted for the better understanding of flooding responsive mechanisms using flooding-tolerant mutant and abscisic acid (ABA)-treated soybean. A total of 146 proteins were usually altered at the early stage of flooding. Proteins related to protein synthesis such as nascent polypeptide-related complex and chaperonin 20, and RNA regulation-associated proteins were up-regulated both at protein and mRNA expression. However, these identified proteins at early stage of flooding were not meaningfully altered. This study suggested that proteins associated with protein synthesis and RNA regulation can influence in triggering tolerance to flooding stress [195]. Therefore, proteomic approaches can be used to understand the response mechanism to drought and flooding stress at the initial stage of soybean growth.

4. Improvement of soybean tolerance to drought and flooding stress

4.1. Breeding objectives and progress of conventional breeding

The objective of soybean breeding programs is to develop cultivars with enhanced yield (more pods/plant, more seeds/pod, 100-seed weight), seed composition (high protein and oil contents), shattering resistance and tolerance to abiotic and biotic stress. Many important agronomic traits (qualitative or simply inherited) are incorporated into commercial cultivar through conventional breeding. As drought and flooding are complex quantitative traits, breeders face difficulties to improve these traits through conventional breeding. Moreover, conventional breeding is tedious, labour extensive, requires a considerable time (8–9 years) and a large amount of space for evaluation. For example, in China, Jindou 21 is an excellent example of drought-tolerant cultivar developed through selective breeding. Initially, Lin Xian White (higher drought tolerance, low yield soybean cultivar) was crossed with Jindou 2 (drought tolerant and high yield).

After six generations, the resulting drought line was selected and further crossed with jindou14. Finally, Jindou 21 was developed after 7 years of selection in arid region of western Shanxi and depicted increased yield under water stress [196]. Xu et al. also identified 463 Chinese strains having high level of drought tolerance through breeding. These strains could be used as a potential source for enhancing drought resistance in soybean [197]. Development of RILs population for flooding tolerance is a long and tedious process. For example, in soybean, to develop F7 population by crossing S992281 X PI4081051 (high yield, flooding tolerant) via single-seed descent method requires 7 years. Hence, conventional breeding approach is less useful [179].

4.2. QTL mapping and marker-assisted selection

To deal with complex nature of drought and flooding, marker-assisted selection to identify QTL can be used as a promising approach. Time consuming phenotypic characterization of large population to get an effective QTL is a major challenge to improve agronomic traits associated with drought and flooding tolerance. If molecular markers are closely linked to the target QTL, it would be possible to transfer character into commercial cultivar through marker-assisted breeding. Marker-assisted selection can be effectively used in soybean having high linkage disequilibrium (low recombinant frequency) [198]. For example, four QTLs associated with root morphology were detected by using 629 SSR markers, indicating that fibrous roots QTL may be related with drought tolerance and seed yield in soybean [144]. In another study, three QTLs for flooding tolerance were detected using 360 SSR markers in soybean. Among three QTLs, one major QTL exhibited large impact on flooding tolerance environments [178].

4.3. Genetic engineering

Genetic engineering in the twenty-first century is a perquisite tool in cell and molecular biology that will provide additional approaches for genetic modification by overexpression or gene silencing, protein sub-cellular localization, transposon mutagenesis and promoter characterization for permitting the development of novel and genetically diverse genotypes. These techniques have become profound strategies in soybean breeding which provide unique chances to modify the genetic makeup of soybean. Recent advancement in genetic mapping and the identification of new drought and flooding stress-responsive genes from various organisms allow researchers to modify plants using several genetic strategies. Genetic transformation in soybean was first reported in 1988 [199, 200], but the stable transformation of soybeans is still a challenging task. Several studies reported on soybean transformation by Agrobacterium-mediated transformation and particle bombardment methods [201, 202]. Both approaches have been used successfully for genetic transformation of soybean. The success is mainly dependent on the efficient delivery of transforming DNA and the recovery of transgenic lines from a transformed cell. Transgenic soybean expressing GMFDL19 gene enhanced tolerance towards drought stress [159] .

4.4. Other new breeding techniques

Over the past 20 years, several new breeding techniques have been developed and are being implemented to facilitate breeding for the crop improvement. New breeding techniques (NBTs) give the ability to accurately modify DNA by editing DNA and genes on or off. Gene or genome editing including CRISPR/Cas9 is a broad category that offers an inexpensive, quick and easy technique to manipulate DNA and lessen the time and effort as compared to traditional breeding. Now-a-days, researchers are working on CRISPR/Cas9-edited versions to improve the different crops such as soybeans, rice, corn, canola and wheat with new traits like drought and flooding resistance and higher yields. Recently, various new plant breeding techniques such as zinc finger nuclease (ZFN) technology, acetate-mediated approach, oligonucleotide-directed mutagenesis (ODM), RNA-dependent DNA methylation (RdDM), cisgenesis, intragenesis, grafting (on GM rootstock) and reverse breeding allow the faster and more efficient improvement of crop varieties.

4.5. Agronomic practices to mitigate the effects of water stress

Agronomic practices can be mitigated the adverse effects of drought and flooding stresses by adopting various strategies. Seed priming is an effective and pragmatic technique to mitigate drought in which seeds are moderately hydrated. In this technique, germination rate, germination percentage and germination uniformity of primed seed increased [11, 203]. This approach has been useful to counteract the effects of drought stress in a range of crop species. Foliar application of plant growth regulators is another technique for improving growth against drought stress. Exogenously applied abscisic acid, uniconazole and brassinolide increased yields both under well-watered and drought conditions in soybean. Plant growth regulator treatments meaningfully increased water potential and chlorophyll contents under water stress conditions [204]. Traditional irrigation system causes >50% loss of irrigated water because of uncovered and unlined ditches. Therefore, a well-managed pipe system is required to avoid losses from traditional irrigation system as it can enhance the conveyance efficiency >90% [205]. Mulching involving covering of soil by using straw or plastic sheets, is another best strategy to retain moisture in soil. For instance, in China, soybean yield increased up to 23.4 and 50.6% by using mulching along with hole sowing and row sowing, respectively [206].

Several management practices have been tried to overcome completely or partially flooding injuries. Flooding induces nitrogen deficiencies resulting in a significant decrease in the uptake of nitrogen. As a result, yellowing of leaves occurred following 2–3 days of flooding. It has been reported that the application of nitrogen fertilizer i.e. polymer-coated urea (PCU) is effective to reduce nitrogen loss and recover flood damage in corn. It also helps to overcome oxygen deficiency in response to flooding stress preferentially [207]. Hypoxia also reduces the capacity of plant to absorb potassium (K). K plays a vital role in alleviating both biotic and abiotic stresses [208]. Indeed, K^+ ions are involved in detoxification of ammonium and ammonia [209], promoting photosynthesis which helps plant recovery and nutrient uptake. Foliar and soil applications oxygen-containing fertilizers lessen the drastic effects of flooding stress [210]. For example, under flooding, oxygen-containing fertilizers considerably retained chlorophyll content and biomass in Italian basil [211].

Under flooding stress, 1-aminocyclopropane-1-carboxylate (ACC) synthase enzyme along with several stress proteins were synthesized [212].The stressed plant consequently produces more ACC in their roots. In roots, ACC cannot be converted into ethylene due to insufficient oxygen. This ACC transferred from roots to shoots converting ACC to ethylene (sufficient oxygen environment) in shoots [213]. In soybean, phytohormone indole acetic acid (IAA) prompts the production of ethylene which prevents the inhibitory effects of high IAA on root growth [214]. Elevation in ethylene production by waterlogged plants results in wilting, necrosis, chlorosis and reduced biomass yield. The application of ACC deaminase-producing plant growth-promoting rhizobacteria (PGPR) can protect plants from these damages [215, 216]. PGPR produce ACC deaminase, which converts ACC into α-ketobutyrate and ammonia, thus reducing the levels of ethylene under water stress conditions. A combination of PGPRs, along with arbuscular mycorrhizal (AM) fungi, including ACC deaminase-producing bacteria, *Pseudomonas, Azospirillum, Rhizobium* and *Bradyrhizobium*, could be a novel step in the alleviation of flooding-impacted plants.

5. Conclusions

Water stress has become major abiotic limitation factor on soybean production under warming climate. To combat drought and flooding stress, there is need to explore the resilient genetic resources and their utilization in breeding program. With the advancement in transcriptomics, proteomics, metabolomics, structural genomics and epigenetics, the production of soybean can be enhanced under water stress by integrating all disciplines. Recent advances in breeding system and agronomic practices will offer an opportunity for significant and predictable incremental improvements in soybean under water stress.

Acknowledgements

This work is supported by the National Key R & D Program for Crop Breeding (2016YF D0100201), the Natural Science Foundation of China (31571691, 31771821), the MOE Program for Changjiang Scholars and Innovative Research Team in University (IRT_17R55), and the Jiangsu JCIC-MCP program.

Author details

Tuanjie Zhao*, Muqadas Aleem and Ripa Akter Sharmin

*Address all correspondence to: tjzhao@njau.edu.cn

Key Laboratory of Biology and Genetics and Breeding for Soybean, National Center for Soybean Improvement, Ministry of Agriculture, State Key Laboratory of Crop Genetics and Germplasm Enhancement, Nanjing Agricultural University, Nanjing, China

References

[1] Wilcox JR. World distribution and trade of soybean. In: Boerma HG, Specht JE, editors. Soybeans: Improvement, Production, and Uses. Vol. 16. Agronomy Monographs. 3rd ed. Madison, WI, USA: ASA-CSSA-SSSA; 2004. pp. 1-14

[2] Koberg M, Abu-Much R, Gedanken A. Optimization of bio-diesel production from soybean and wastes of cooked oil: Combining dielectric microwave irradiation and a SrO catalyst. Bioresource Technology. 2011;**102**:1073-1078. DOI: 10.1016/j.biortech.2010.08.055

[3] Jooyandeh H. Soy products as healthy and functional foods. Middle-East Journal of Scientific Research. 2011;**7**:71-80

[4] Goldsmith PD. Economics of soybean production, marketing and utilization. In: Johnson LA, White PJ, Galloway R, editors. Soybeans: Chemistry, Production Processing and Utilization. Urbana: AOCS Press; 2008. pp. 117-150

[5] Boyer JS. Plant productivity and environment. Science. 1982;**218**:443-448. DOI: 10.1126/science.218.4571.443

[6] Thomas CD, Cameron A, Green RE, Bakkenes M, Beaumont LJ, Collingham YC, et al. Extinction risk from climate change. Nature. 2004;**427**:145-148. DOI: 10.1038/nature02121

[7] Ahmed F, Rafii M, Ismail MR, Juraimi AS, Rahim H, Asfaliza R, et al. Waterlogging tolerance of crops: Breeding, mechanism of tolerance, molecular approaches, and future prospects. BioMed Research International. 2013;**2013**:1-10. DOI: 10.1155/2013/963525

[8] Valliyodan B, Nguyen HT. Understanding regulatory networks and engineering for enhanced drought tolerance in plants. Current Opinion in Plant Biology. 2006;**9**:189-195. DOI: 10.1016/j.pbi.2006.01.019

[9] Szilagyi L. Influence of drought on seed yield components in common bean. Bulgarian Journal of Plant Physiology 2003;**2003**:320-330

[10] Hirt H, Shinozaki K. Topics in Current Genetics, Plant Responses to Abiotic Stress. Heildelberg: Springer Science & Business Media Berlin; 2004

[11] Kaya MD, Okçu G, Atak M, Çıkılı Y, Kolsarıcı Ö. Seed treatments to overcome salt and drought stress during germination in sunflower (*Helianthus annuus* L.). European Journal of Agronomy. 2006;**24**:291-295. DOI: 10.1016/j.eja.2005.08.001

[12] Okçu G, Kaya MD, Atak M. Effects of salt and drought stresses on germination and seedling growth of pea (*Pisum sativum* L.). Turkish Journal of Agriculture and Forestry. 2005;**29**:237-242

[13] Zeid I, Shedeed Z. Response of alfalfa to putrescine treatment under drought stress. Biologia Plantarum. 2006;**50**:635-640. DOI: 10.1007/s10535-006-0099-9

[14] Boyer JS. Subcellular mechanisms of plant response to low water potential. Agricultural Water Management. 1983;**7**:239-248. DOI: 10.1016/0378-3774(83)90087-2

[15] Turner NC, Wright GC, Siddique K. Adaptation of grain legumes (pulses) to water-limited environments. Advances in Agronomy. 2001;**71**:193-231. DOI: 10.1016/S0065-2113[01]71015-2

[16] Boerma HR, Specht JE. Soybeans: improvement, production and uses. Agronomy Monographs. Vol. 16, 3rd ed. Madison, WI, USA: ASA-CSSA-SSSA; 2004

[17] Purcell LC, Specht JE. Physiological traits for ameliorating drought stress. In: Boerma HG, Specht JE, editors. Soybeans: Improvement, Production, and Uses. Vol. 16. Agronomy Monographs. 3rd ed. Madison, WI, USA: ASA-CSSA-SSSA; 2004. pp. 559-620. DOI: 10.2134/agronmonogr16.3ed.c12

[18] Kavar T, Maras M, Kidrič M, Šuštar-Vozlič J, Meglič V. Identification of genes involved in the response of leaves of *Phaseolus vulgaris* to drought stress. Molecular Breeding. 2008;**21**:159-172. DOI: 10.1007/s11032-007-9116-8

[19] Nguyen HT, Babu RC, Blum A. Breeding for drought resistance in rice: Physiology and molecular genetics considerations. Crop Science. 1997;**37**:1426-1434. DOI: 10.2135/cropsci1997.0011183X003700050002x

[20] Mittler R. Abiotic stress, the field environment and stress combination. Trends in Plant Science. 2006;**11**:15-19. DOI: 10.1016/j.tplants.2005.11.002

[21] Valliyodan B, Van Toai TT, Alves JD, de Fátima P, Goulart P, Lee JD, Fritschi FB, et al. Expression of root-related transcription factors associated with flooding tolerance of soybean (*Glycine max*). International Journal of Molecular Sciences. 2014;**15**:17622-17643. DOI: 10.3390/ijms151017622

[22] Kokubun M. Genetic and cultural improvement of soybean for waterlogged conditions in Asia. Field Crops Research. 2013;**152**:3-7. DOI: 10.1016/j.fcr.2012.09.022

[23] Kosturkova G, Todorova R, Sakthivelu G, Akitha Devi M, Giridhar P, Rajasekaran T, et al. Response of bulgarian and indian soybean genotypes to drought and water deficiency in field and laboratory conditions. General and Applied Plant Physiology. 2008;**34**:239-250

[24] Rasaei B, Ghobadi M-E, Khas-Amiri M, Ghobadi M. Effect of osmotic potential on germination and seedling characteristics of soybean seeds. International Journal of Agriculture and Crop Sciences. 2013;**5**:1265

[25] Hossain MM, Liu X, Qi X, Lam H-M, Zhang J. Differences between soybean genotypes in physiological response to sequential soil drying and rewetting. The Crop Journal. 2014;**2**:366-380

[26] Hossain MM, Lam H-M, Zhang J. Responses in gas exchange and water status between drought-tolerant and-susceptible soybean genotypes with ABA application. The Crop Journal. 2015;**3**:500-506. DOI: 10.1016/j.cj.2014.08.001

[27] Fenta BA, Beebe SE, Kunert KJ, Burridge JD, Barlow KM, Lynch JP, et al. Field phenotyping of soybean roots for drought stress tolerance. Agronomy. 2014;**4**:418-435. DOI: 10.3390/Agronomy4030418

[28] Sepanlo N, Talebi R, Rokhzadi A, Mohammadi H. Morphological and physiological behavior in soybean (*Glycine max*) genotypes to drought stress implemented at pre-and post-anthesis stages. Acta Biologica Szegediensis. 2014;**58**:109-113

[29] Kobraei S, Etminan A, Mohammadi R, Kobraee S. Effects of drought stress on yield and yield components of soybean. Annals of Biological Research. 2011;**2**:504-509

[30] Kobraee S, Shamsi K, Rasekhi B. Soybean production under water deficit conditions. Annals of Biological Research. 2011;**2**:423-434

[31] Prince SJ, Murphy M, Mutava RN, Durnell LA, Valliyodan B, Shannon JG, et al. Root xylem plasticity to improve water use and yield in water-stressed soybean. Journal of Experimental Botany. 2017;**68**:2027-2036. DOI: 10.1093/jxb/erw472

[32] Chowdhury J, Karim M, Khaliq Q, Solaiman A, Ahmed J. Screening of soybean (*Glycine max* L.) genotypes under water stress condition. Bangladesh Journal of Agricultural Research. 2016;**41**:441-450. DOI: 10.3329/bjar.v41i3.29716

[33] Shimamura S, Mochizuki T, Nada Y, Fukuyama M. Formation and function of secondary aerenchyma in hypocotyl, roots and nodules of soybean (*Glycine max*) under flooded conditions. Plant and Soil. 2003;**251**:351-359. DOI: 10.1023/A:1023036720537

[34] Henshaw T, Gilbert R, Scholberg J, Sinclair T. Soya bean (*Glycine max* L. Merr.) genotype response to early-season flooding: I. Root and nodule development. Journal of Agronomy and Crop Science. 2007;**193**:177-188. DOI: 10.1111/j.1439-037X.2007.00257.x

[35] Henshaw T, Gilbert R, Scholberg J, Sinclair T. Soya bean (*Glycine max* L. Merr.) genotype response to early-season flooding: II. Aboveground growth and biomass. Journal of Agronomy and Crop Science. 2007;**193**:189-197. DOI: 10.1111/j.1439-037X.2007.00258.x

[36] Oh K-W, Lim S-G, Kim S-R, Ko J-M, Han W-Y, Kim H-T, et al. Flooding affects root morphology and photosynthesis in soybean (*Glycine max* [L.] Merr.). Journal of the Korean Society of the Crop Science. 2008;**120**:1

[37] Sakazono S, Nagata T, Matsuo R, Kajihara S, Watanabe M, Ishimoto M, et al. Variation in root development response to flooding among 92 soybean lines during early growth stages. Plant Production Science. 2014;**17**:228-236. DOI: 10.1626/pps.17.228

[38] Borella J, do Amarante L, de Oliveira, DDC, de Oliveira, ACB, Braga EJB. Waterlogging-induced changes in fermentative metabolism in roots and nodules of soybean genotypes. Scientia Agricola 2014;**71**:499-508. DOI: 10.1590/0103-9016-2014-0044

[39] Nguyen VL, Binh VT, Hoang DT, Mochizuki T, Nguyen VL. Genotypic variation in morphological and physiological response of soybean to waterlogging at flowering stage. International Journal of Agricultural Science Research. 2015;**4**:150-157

[40] Suematsu K, Abiko T, Nguyen VL, Mochizuki T. Phenotypic variation in root development of 162 soybean accessions under hypoxia condition at the seedling stage. Plant Production Science. 2017;**20**:323-335. DOI: 10.1080/1343943X.2017.1334511

[41] Oosterhuis D, Scott H, Hampton R, Wullschleger S. Physiological responses of two soybean (*Glycine max* [L.] Merr) cultivars to short-term flooding. Environmental and Experimental Botany. 1990;**30**:85-92

[42] Colmer T, Voesenek L. Flooding tolerance: Suites of plant traits in variable environments. Functional Plant Biology. 2009;**36**:665-681. DOI: 10.1016/0098-8472[90]90012-S

[43] van Veen H, Mustroph A, Barding GA, Vergeer-van Eijk M, Welschen-Evertman RA, Pedersen O, et al. Two Rumex species from contrasting hydrological niches regulate flooding tolerance through distinct mechanisms. The Plant Cell. 2013;**25**:4691-6707. DOI: 10.1105/tpc.113.119016

[44] Bailey-Serres J, Voesenek L. Flooding stress: Acclimations and genetic diversity. Annual Review of Plant Biology. 2008;**59**:313-339. DOI: 10.1146/annurev.arplant.59.032607.092752

[45] Bengough AG, McKenzie B, Hallett P, Valentine T. Root elongation, water stress, and mechanical impedance: A review of limiting stresses and beneficial root tip traits. Journal of Experimental Botany. 2011;**62**:59-68. DOI: 10.1093/jxb/erq350

[46] Fehr WR, Caviness CE, Burmood D, Pennington J. Stage of development descriptions for soybeans, *Glycine max* [L.] Merrill. Crop Science. 1971;**11**:929-931

[47] Tanaka N, Kato M, Tomioka R, Kurata R, Fukao Y, Aoyama T, et al. Characteristics of a root hair-less line of *Arabidopsis thaliana* under physiological stresses. Journal of Experimental Botany. 2014;**65**:1497-1512. DOI: 10.1093/jxb/eru014

[48] Vadez V. Root hydraulics: The forgotten side of roots in drought adaptation. Field Crops Research. 2014;**165**:15-24. DOI: 10.1016/j.fcr.2014.03.017

[49] Serraj R, Bona S, Purcell LC, Sinclair TR. Nitrogen accumulation and nodule activity of field-grown 'Jackson'soybean in response to water deficits. Field Crops Research. 1997;**52**:109-116. DOI: 10.1016/S0378-4290[96]01068-4

[50] Prince SJ, Murphy M, Mutava RN, Zhang Z, Nguyen N, Kim YH, et al. Evaluation of high yielding soybean germplasm under water limitation. Journal of Integrative Plant Biology. 2016;**58**:475-491. DOI: 10.1111/jipb.12378

[51] Garay A, Wilhelm W. Root system characteristics of two soybean isolines undergoing water stress conditions. Agronomy Journal. 1983;**75**:973-977. DOI: 10.2134/agronj1983.00021962007500060026x

[52] Liu Y, Gai J-Y, Lu H, Wang Y-J, Chen S-Y. Identification of drought tolerant germplasm and inheritance and QTL mapping of related root traits in soybean (*Glycine max* [L.] Merr). Acta Genetica Sinica. 2005;**32**:855-863

[53] He J, Jin Y, Y-L D, Wang T, Turner NC, Yang R-P, et al. Genotypic variation in yield, yield components, root morphology and architecture, in soybean in relation to water and phosphorus supply. Frontiers in Plant Science. 2017;**8**:1499. DOI: 10.3389/fpls.2017.01499

[54] Liu F, Andersen MN, Jensen CR. Loss of pod set caused by drought stress is associated with water status and ABA content of reproductive structures in soybean. Functional Plant Biology. 2003;**30**:271-280. DOI: 10.1071/FP02185

[55] Stolf-Moreira R, Medri M, Neumaier N, Lemos N, Pimenta J, Tobita S, et al. Soybean physiology and gene expression during drought. Genetics and Molecular Research. 2010;**9**:1946-1956. DOI: 10.4238/vol9-4gmr851

[56] Laan P, Berrevoets M, Lythe S, Armstrong W, Blom C. Root morphology and aerenchyma formation as indicators of the flood-tolerance of *Rumex* species. The Journal of Ecology. 1989;**77**:693-703. DOI: 10.2307/2260979

[57] Smirnoff N, Crawford R. Variation in the structure and response to flooding of root aerenchyma in some wetland plants. Annals of Botany. 1983;**51**:237-249. DOI: 10.1093/oxfordjournals.aob.a086462

[58] Kawai M, Samarajeewa P, Barrero R, Nishiguchi M, Uchimiya H. Cellular dissection of the degradation pattern of cortical cell death during aerenchyma formation of rice roots. Planta. 1998;**204**:277-287. DOI: 10.1007/s004250050257

[59] Seago JRJL, Marsh LC, Stevens KJ, Soukup A, Votrubova O, Enstone DE. A re-examination of the root cortex in wetland flowering plants with respect to aerenchyma. Annals of Botany. 2005;**96**:565-579. DOI: 10.1093/aob/mci211

[60] Drew MC, He C-J, Morgan PW. Programmed cell death and aerenchyma formation in roots. Trends in Plant Science. 2000;**5**:123-127. DOI: 10.1016/S1360-1385(00)01570-3

[61] Steffens B, Kovalev A, Gorb SN, Sauter M. Emerging roots alter epidermal cell fate through mechanical and reactive oxygen species signaling. The Plant Cell. 2012;**24**:3296-3306. DOI: 10.1105/tpc.112.101790

[62] Thomas A, Guerreiro S, Sodek L. Aerenchyma formation and recovery from hypoxia of the flooded root system of nodulated soybean. Annals of Botany. 2005;**96**:1191-1198. DOI: 10.1093/aob/mci272

[63] Bacanamwo M, Purcell LC. Soybean dry matter and N accumulation responses to flooding stress, N sources and hypoxia. Journal of Experimental Botany. 1999;**50**:689-696. DOI: 10.1093/jexbot/50.334.689

[64] Shimamura S, Yamamoto R, Nakamura T, Shimada S, Komatsu S. Stem hypertrophic lenticels and secondary aerenchyma enable oxygen transport to roots of soybean in flooded soil. Annals of Botany. 2010;**106**:277-284. DOI: 10.1093/aob/mcq123

[65] Vidoz ML, Loreti E, Mensuali A, Alpi A, Perata P. Hormonal interplay during adventitious root formation in flooded tomato plants. The Plant Journal. 2010;**63**:551-562. DOI: 10.1111/j.1365-313X.2010.04262.x

[66] Tamang BG, Magliozzi JO, Maroof MS, Fukao T. Physiological and transcriptomic characterization of submergence and reoxygenation responses in soybean seedlings. Plant, cell & Environment. 2014;**37**:2350-2365. DOI: 10.1111/pce.12277

[67] Evans DE. Aerenchyma formation. New Phytologist. 2004;**161**:35-49. DOI: 10.1046/j.1469-8137.2003.00907.x

[68] Phukan UJ, Mishra S, Timbre K, Luqman S, Shukla RK. *Mentha arvensis* exhibit better adaptive characters in contrast to *Mentha piperita* when subjugated to sustained waterlogging stress. Protoplasma. 2014;**251**:603-614. DOI: 10.1007/s00709-013-0561-4

[69] Makbul S, Guler NS, Durmus N, Guven S. Changes in anatomical and physiological parameters of soybean under drought stress. Turkish Journal of Botany. 2011;**35**:369-377. DOI: 10.3906/bot-1002-7

[70] Hernández JA, Ferrer MA, Jiménez A, Barceló AR, Sevilla F. Antioxidant systems and O2.−/H2O2 production in the apoplast of pea leaves. Its relation with salt-induced necrotic lesions in minor veins. Plant Physiology. 2001;**127**:817-831. DOI: 10.1104/pp.010188

[71] Türkan İ, Bor M, Özdemir F, Koca H. Differential responses of lipid peroxidation and antioxidants in the leaves of drought-tolerant *P. acutifolius* Gray and drought-sensitive *P. vulgaris* L. subjected to polyethylene glycol mediated water stress. Plant Science. 2005;**168**:223-231. DOI: 10.1016/j.plantsci.2004.07.032

[72] Clement M, Lambert A, Herouart D, Boncompagni E. Identification of new up-regulated genes under drought stress in soybean nodules. Gene. 2008;**426**:15-22. DOI: 10.1016/j.gene. 2008.08.016

[73] Creissen GP, Mullineaux PM. The molecular biology of the ascorbate-glutathione cycle in higher plants. In: Inzé D, Montgan MV, editors. Oxidative Stress in Plants. UK: Taylor & Francis; 2002. pp. 247-270

[74] Aroca R, Irigoyen JJ, Sánchez-Díaz M. Drought enhances maize chilling tolerance. II. Photosynthetic traits and protective mechanisms against oxidative stress. Physiologia Plantarum. 2003;**117**:540-549. DOI: 10.1034/j.1399-3054.2003.00065.x

[75] Masoumi H, Masoumi M, Darvish F, Daneshian J, Nourmohammadi G, Habibi D. Change in several antioxidant enzymes activity and seed yield by water deficit stress in soybean (*Glycine max* L.) cultivars. Notulae Botanicae Horti Agrobotanici Cluj-Napoca. 2010;**38**: 86-94. DOI: 10.15835/nbha3834936

[76] Else MA, Coupland D, Dutton L, Jackson MB. Decreased root hydraulic conductivity reduces leaf water potential, initiates stomatal closure and slows leaf expansion in flooded plants of castor oil (*Ricinus communis*) despite diminished delivery of ABA from the roots to shoots in xylem sap. Physiologia Plantarum. 2001;**111**:46-54. DOI: 10.1034/j.1399-3054.2001.1110107.x

[77] Jackson M, Hall K. Early stomatal closure in waterlogged pea plants is mediated by abscisic acid in the absence of foliar water deficits. Plant, Cell & Environment. 1987;**10**:121-130. DOI: 10.1111/1365-3040.ep11602085

[78] Malik AI, Colmer TD, Lambers H, Schortemeyer M. Changes in physiological and morphological traits of roots and shoots of wheat in response to different depths of waterlogging. Functional Plant Biology. 2001;**28**:1121-1131. DOI: 10.1071/PP01089

[79] Boru G, Vantoai T, Alves J, Hua D, Knee M. Responses of soybean to oxygen deficiency and elevated root-zone carbon dioxide concentration. Annals of Botany. 2003;**91**:447-453. DOI: 10.1093/aob/mcg040

[80] Fukao T, Xu K, Ronald PC, Bailey-Serres J. A variable cluster of ethylene response factor–like genes regulates metabolic and developmental acclimation responses to submergence in rice. The Plant Cell. 2006;**18**:2021-2034. DOI: 10.1105/tpc.106.043000

[81] Mommer L, Pons TL, Wolters-Arts M, Venema JH, Visser EJ. Submergence-induced morphological, anatomical, and biochemical responses in a terrestrial species affect gas diffusion resistance and photosynthetic performance. Plant Physiology. 2005;**139**:497-508. DOI: 10.1104/pp.105.064725

[82] Jackson MB, Attwood PA. Roots of willow [*Salix viminalis* L.] show marked tolerance to oxygen shortage in flooded soils and in solution culture. Plant and Soil. 1996;**187**:37-45

[83] Yordanova RY, Christov KN, Popova LP. Antioxidative enzymes in barley plants subjected to soil flooding. Environmental and Experimental Botany. 2004;**51**:93-101. DOI: 10.1016/S0098-8472[03]00063-7

[84] Vieira RD, Tekrony D, Egli D. Effect of drought and defoliation stress in the field on soybean seed germination and vigor. Crop Science. 1992;**32**:471-475

[85] Dornbos Jr D, Mullen R. Influence of stress during soybean seed fill on seed weight, germination, and seedling growth rate. Canadian Journal of Plant Science. 1991;**71**:373-383. DOI: 10.4141/cjps91-052

[86] Maleki A, Naderi A, Naseri R, Fathi A, Bahamin S, Maleki R. Physiological performance of soybean cultivars under drought stress. Bulletin of environment, pharmacology and. Life Sciences. 2013;**2**:38-44

[87] Guffy R, Hesketh J, Nelson R, Bernard R. Seed growth rate, growth duration, and yield in soybean. Biotronics: Reports of Biotron Institute, Kyushu University. 1991;**20**:19-30

[88] Maryam A, Nasreen SA. Review: Water logging effects on morphological, anatomical, physiological and biochemical attributes of food and cash crops. International Journal of Water Resources and Environmental Sciences. 2012;**1**:113-120. DOI: 10.5829/idosi.ijwres.2012.1.4.11119

[89] Yaklich RW, Abdul-Baki AA. Variability in metabolism of individual axes of soybean seeds and its relationship to vigor. Crop Science. 1975;**15**:424-426. DOI: 10.2135/cropsci1975.0011183X001500030042x

[90] Wuebker EF, Mullen RE, Koehler K. Flooding and temperature effects on soybean germination. Crop Science. 2001;**41**:1857-1861. DOI: 10.2135/cropsci2001.1857

[91] Sayama T, Nakazaki T, Ishikawa G, Yagasaki K, Yamada N, Hirota N, et al. QTL analysis of seed-flooding tolerance in soybean (*Glycine max* [L.] Merr.). Plant Science. 2009;**176**:514-521. DOI: 10.1016/j.plantsci.2009.01.007

[92] Manavalan LP, Guttikonda SK, Phan Tran L-S, Nguyen HT. Physiological and molecular approaches to improve drought resistance in soybean. Plant and Cell Physiology. 2009;**50**:1260-1276. DOI: 10.1093/pcp/pcp082

[93] Desclaux D, Huynh TT, Roumet P. Identification of soybean plant characteristics that indicate the timing of drought stress. Crop Science. 2000;**40**:716-722. DOI: 10.2135/cropsci2000.403716x

[94] Jackson M, Ricard B. Physiology, biochemistry and molecular biology of plant root systems subjected to flooding of the soil. In: Visser EJW, de Kroon H, editors. Root Ecology. Heidelberg: Springer-Verlag; 2003. pp. 193-213. DOI: 10.1007/978-3-662-09784-78

[95] Jackson MB, Drew MC, Kozlowski T. Effect of flooding on growth and metabolism of herbaceous plants. In: Kozlowski TT, editor. Flooding and Plant Growth. New York: Academic Press; 1984. pp. 47-128. DOI: 10.1093/aob/mcg014

[96] Kramer PJ. Causes of injury to plants resulting from flooding of the soil. Plant Physiology. 1951;**26**:722. DOI: 10.1104/pp.26.4.722

[97] Sallam A, Scott H. Effects of prolonged flooding on soybeans during early vegetative growth. Soil Science. 1987;**144**:61-66. DOI: 10.1080/01904168709363593

[98] Gladish DK, Xu J, Niki T. Apoptosis-like programmed cell death occurs in procambium and ground meristem of pea (*Pisum sativum*) root tips exposed to sudden flooding. Annals of Botany. 2006;**97**:895-902. DOI: 10.1093/aob/mcl040

[99] Nanjo Y, Nakamura T, Komatsu S. Identification of indicator proteins associated with flooding injury in soybean seedlings using label-free quantitative proteomics. Journal of Proteome Research. 2013;**12**:4785-4798. DOI: 10.1021/pr4002349

[100] Subbaiah CC, Sachs MM. Molecular and cellular adaptations of maize to flooding stress. Annals of Botany. 2003;**91**:119-127. DOI: 10.1093/aob/mcf210

[101] Ohashi Y, Nakayama N, Saneoka H, Mohapatra PK, Fujita K. Differences in the responses of stem diameter and pod thickness to drought stress during the grain filling stage in soybean plants. Acta Physiologiae Plantarum. 2009;**31**:271-277. DOI: 10.1007/s11738-008-0229-4

[102] Nobuyasu H, Liu S, Adu-Gyamfi J, Mohapatra P, Fujita K. Variation in the export of 13 C and 15 N from soybean leaf: The effects of nitrogen application and sink removal. Plant and Soil. 2003;**253**:331-339. DOI: 10.1023/A:1024836600725

[103] Westgate M, Peterson C. Flower and pod development in water-deficient soybeans (*Glycine max* L. Merr). Journal of Experimental Botany. 1993;**44**:109-117. DOI: 10.1093/jxb/44.1.109

[104] Ekhtiari S, Kobraee S, Shamsi K. Soybean yield under water deficit conditions. Journal of biodiversity and environment. Science. 2013;**3**:46-52

[105] VanToai T, Beuerlein A, Schmitthenner S, St Martin S. Genetic variability for flooding tolerance in soybeans. Crop Science. 1994;**34**:1112-1115. DOI: 10.2135/cropsci1994.0011183X003400040051x

[106] Linkemer G, Board JE, Musgrave ME. Waterlogging effects on growth and yield components in late-planted soybean. Crop Science. 1998;**38**:1576-1584. DOI: 10.2135/cropsci1998.0011183X003800060028x

[107] Sullivan M, VanToai T, Fausey N, Beuerlein J, Parkinson R, Soboyejo A. Evaluating on-farm flooding impacts on soybean. Crop Science. 2001;**41**:93-100. DOI: 10.2135/cropsci2001.41193x

[108] Griffin JL, Saxton AM. Response of solid-seeded soybean to flood irrigation. II. Flood duration. Agronomy Journal. 1988;**80**:885-888. DOI: 10.2134/agronj1988.00021962008000060009x

[109] Schöffel ER, Saccol AV, Manfron PA, Medeiros SLP. Excesso hídrico sobre os componentes do rendimento da cultura da soja. Ciência Rural. 2001;**31**:7-12. DOI: 10.1590/S0103-84782001000100002

[110] Rhine MD, Stevens G, Shannon G, Wrather A, Sleper D. Yield and nutritional responses to waterlogging of soybean cultivars. Irrigation Science. 2010;**28**:135-142. DOI: 10.1007/s00271-009-0168-x

[111] Neumaier N, Farias JR, Nepomuceno AL. Índice de tolerância à seca em quatro cultivares de soja. In: Sociedade Brasileira de Agrometeorologia, Anais. Congresso Brasileiro de Agrometeorologia. Campina Grande, PB; 1995. p. 80-82

[112] Valliyodan B, Ye H, Song L, Murphy M, Shannon JG, Nguyen HT. Genetic diversity and genomic strategies for improving drought and waterlogging tolerance in soybeans. Journal of Experimental Botany. 2016;**68**:1835-1849. DOI: 10.1093/jxb/erw433

[113] Thu NBA, Nguyen QT, Hoang XLT, Thao NP, Tran L-SP. Evaluation of drought tolerance of the Vietnamese soybean cultivars provides potential resources for soybean production and genetic engineering. BioMed Research International. 2014;**2014**:1-9. DOI: 10.1155/2014/809736

[114] VanToai TT, Hoa TTC, Hue NTN, Nguyen HT, Shannon JG, Rahman MA. Flooding tolerance of soybean (*Glycine max* [L.] Merr.) germplasm from Southeast Asia under field and screen-house environments. The Open Agriculture Journal. 2010;**4**:38-46. DOI: 10.2174/1874331501004010038

[115] Koo SC, Kim HT, Kang BK, Lee YH, Oh KW, Kim HY, et al. Screening of flooding tolerance in soybean germplam collection. Korean Journal of Breeding Science. 2014;**46**:129-135. DOI: 10.9787/KJBS.2014.46.2.129

[116] Seversike TM, Sermons SM, Sinclair TR, Carter TE, Rufty TW. Physiological properties of a drought-resistant wild soybean genotype: Transpiration control with soil drying and expression of root morphology. Plant and Soil. 2014;**374**:359-370. DOI: 10.1007/s11104-013-1757-2

[117] Prince SJ, Song L, Qiu D, dos Santos JVM, Chai C, Joshi T, et al. Genetic variants in root architecture-related genes in a *Glycine soja* accession, a potential resource to improve cultivated soybean. BMC Genomics. 2015;**16**:132. DOI: 10.1186/s12864-015-1334-6

[118] Pathan MS, Lee JD, Shannon JG, Nguyen HT. Recent advances in breeding for drought and salt stress tolerance in soybean. In: Jenks MA, Hasegawa PM, Jain S, editors. Advances in molecular breeding toward drought and salt tolerant crops. Germany: Springer; 2007. pp. 739-773. DOI: 10.1007/978-1-4020-5578-230

[119] Hwang S, King CA, Ray JD, Cregan PB, Chen P, Carter TE, et al. Confirmation of delayed canopy wilting QTLs from multiple soybean mapping populations. Theoretical and Applied Genetics. 2015;**128**:2047-2065. DOI: 10.1007/s00122-015-2566-1

[120] Abdel-Haleem H, Carter TE, Purcell LC, King CA, Ries LL, Chen P, et al. Mapping of quantitative trait loci for canopy-wilting trait in soybean (*Glycine max* L. Merr). Theoretical and Applied Genetics. 2012;**125**:837-846. DOI: 10.1007/s00122-012-1876-9

[121] Charlson DV, Bhatnagar S, King CA, Ray JD, Sneller CH, Carter TE, et al. Polygenic inheritance of canopy wilting in soybean (*Glycine max* [L.] Merr.). Theoretical and Applied Genetics. 2009;**119**:587-594. DOI: 10.1007/s00122-009-1068-4

[122] Bhatnagar S, King CA, Purcell L, Ray JD. Identification and mapping of quantitative trait loci associated with crop responses to water-deficit stress in soybean (*Glycine max* [L.] Merr.). The ASACSSA-SSSA International Annual Meeting Poster Abstract; Salt Lake City, UT, USA. November 6-10, 2005

[123] Specht J, Chase K, Macrander M, Graef G, Chung J, Markwell J, et al. Soybean response to water. Crop Science. 2001;**41**:493-509. DOI: 10.2135/cropsci2001.412493x

[124] Monteros M, Lee G, Missaoui AM, Carter TE, Boerma HR Identification and confirmation of QTL conditioning drought tolerance in Nepalese soybean PI471938. In: The 11th Biennial Conference on the Molecular and Cellular Biology of the Soybean; Lincoln, Nebraska. August 5-8, 2006

[125] Mian M, Ashley D, Boerma H. An additional QTL for water use efficiency in soybean. Crop Science. 1998;**38**:390-393. DOI: 10.2135/cropsci1998.0011183X003800020020x

[126] Mian MA, Bailey MA, Ashley DA, Wells R, Carter TE, Parrott WA, Boerma HR. Molecular markers associated with water use efficiency and leaf ash in soybean. Crop Science. 1996;**36**:1252-1257

[127] Hwang S, King CA, Davies MK, Ray JD, Cregan PB, Purcell LCQTL. Analysis of shoot Ureide and nitrogen concentrations in soybean (*Glycine max* [L.] Merr.). Crop Science. 2013;**53**:2421-2433. DOI: 10.2135/cropsci2012.11.0641

[128] Du W, Wang M, Fu S, Mapping YD. QTLs for seed yield and drought susceptibility index in soybean (*Glycine max* L.) across different environments. Journal of Genetics and Genomics. 2009;**36**:721-731. DOI: 10.1016/S1673-8527[08]60165-4

[129] Anandan A, Anumalla M, Pradhan SK, Ali J. Population structure, diversity and trait association analysis in rice (*Oryza sativa* L.) germplasm for early seedling vigor (ESV) using trait linked SSR markers. PLoS One. 2016;**11**:e0152406. DOI: 10.1371/journal.pone.0152406

[130] Carter Jr TE, De Souza PI, Purcell LC, editors. Recent advances in breeding for drought and aluminum resistance in soybean. In: Proceedings of the World Soybean Conference VI Chicago, IL; August 4, 1999. pp. 4-7. DOI: 10.1007/978-1-4020-5578-230

[131] Aceves-García P, Álvarez-Buylla ER, Garay-Arroyo A, García-Ponce B, Muñoz R, de la Paz Sánchez M. Root architecture diversity and meristem dynamics in different populations of *Arabidopsis thaliana*. Frontiers in Plant Science. 2016;**7**:858. DOI: 10.3389/fpls.2016.00858

[132] Uga Y, Sugimoto K, Ogawa S, Rane J, Ishitani M, Hara N, et al. Control of root system architecture by Deeping rooting 1 increases rice yield under drought conditions. Nature Genetics. 2013;**45**:1097-1102

[133] Pinto RS, Reynolds MP. Common genetic basis for canopy temperature depression under heat and drought stress associated with optimized root distribution in bread wheat. Theoretical and Applied Genetics. 2015;**128**:575-585. DOI: 10.1007/s00122-015-2453-9

[134] Ellsworth PZ, Cousins AB. Carbon isotopes and water use efficiency in C_4 plants. Current Opinion in Plant Biology. 2016;**31**:155-161. DOI: 10.1016/j.pbi.2016.04.006

[135] Tambussi EA, Bort J, Guiamet JJ, Nogués S, Araus JL. The photosynthetic role of ears in C_3 cereals: Metabolism, water use efficiency and contribution to grain yield. Critical Reviews in Plant Sciences. 2007;**26**:1-16

[136] Feller U. Drought stress and carbon assimilation in a warming climate: Reversible and irreversible impacts. Journal of Plant Physiology. 2016;**203**:84-94. DOI: 10.1016/j.jplph.2016.04.002

[137] Tuinstra M, Ejeta G, Goldsbrough P. Evaluation of near-isogenic sorghum lines contrasting for QTL markers associated with drought tolerance. Crop Science. 1998;**38**:835-842

[138] Djekoun A, Planchon C. Water status effect on dinitrogen fixation and photosynthesis in soybean. Agronomy Journal. 1991;**83**:316-322. DOI: 10.2134/agronj1991.00021962008300020011x

[139] Sadras VO, Lake L, Li Y, Farquharson EA, Sutton T. Phenotypic plasticity and its genetic regulation for yield, nitrogen fixation and δ13C in chickpea crops under varying water regimes. Journal of Experimental Botany. 2016;**67**:4339-4351

[140] Sinclair T, Serraj R. Legume nitrogen-fixation and drought. Nature. 1995;**378**:344. DOI: 10.1038/378344a0

[141] Sulieman S, Ha CV, Nasr Esfahani M, Watanabe Y, Nishiyama R, Pham CTB, et al. DT2008: A promising new genetic resource for improved drought tolerance in soybean when solely dependent on symbiotic N2 fixation. BioMed Research International. 2015;**2015**:687213. DOI: 10.1155/2015/687213

[142] Sinclair TR, Messina CD, Beatty A, Samples M. Assessment across the United States of the benefits of altered soybean drought traits. Agronomy Journal. 2010;**102**:475-482. DOI: 10.2134/agronj2009.0195

[143] Specht J, Hume D, Kumudini S. Soybean yield potential – A genetic and physiological perspective. Crop Science. 1999;**39**:1560-1570. DOI: 10.2135/cropsci1999.3961560x

[144] Abdel-Haleem H, Lee GJ, Boerma RH. Identification of QTL for increased fibrous roots in soybean. Theoretical and Applied Genetics. 2011;**122**:935-946. DOI: 10.1007/s00122-010-1500-9

[145] Atkinson JA, Wingen LU, Griffiths M, Pound MP, Gaju O, Foulkes MJ, et al. Phenotyping pipeline reveals major seedling root growth QTL in hexaploid wheat. Journal of Experimental Botany. 2015;**66**:2283-2292. DOI: 10.1093/jxb/erv006

[146] Courtois B, Ahmadi N, Khowaja F, Price AH, Rami J-F, Frouin J, et al. Rice root genetic architecture: Meta-analysis from a drought QTL database. Rice. 2009;**2**:115-128. DOI: 10.1007/s12284-009-9028-9

[147] Giuliani S, Sanguineti MC, Tuberosa R, Bellotti M, Salvi S, Landi P. Root-ABA1, a major constitutive QTL, affects maize root architecture and leaf ABA concentration at different water regimes. Journal of Experimental Botany. 2005;**56**:3061-3070. DOI: 10.1093/jxb/eri303

[148] Manavalan LP, Prince SJ, Musket TA, Chaky J, Deshmukh R, Vuong TD, et al. Identification of novel QTL governing root architectural traits in an interspecific soybean population. PLoS One. 2015;**10**:e0120490. DOI: 10.1371/journal.pone.0120490

[149] Deshmukh RK, Sonah H, Kondawar V, Singh Tomar RS, Deshmukh NK. Identification of meta quantitative trait loci for agronomical traits in rice (*Oryza sativa*). Indian Journal of Genetics and Plant Breeding. 2012;**72**:264-270

[150] Sosnowski O, Charcosset A, Joets J. BioMercator V3: An upgrade of genetic map compilation and quantitative trait loci meta-analysis algorithms. Bioinformatics. 2012;**28**: 2082-2083. DOI: 10.1093/bioinformatics/bts313

[151] Hwang S, King CA, Chen P, Ray JD, Cregan PB, Carter Jr TE, et al. Meta-analysis to refine map position and reduce confidence intervals for delayed-canopy-wilting QTLs in soybean. Molecular Breeding. 2016;**36**:1-14. DOI: 10.1007/s11032-016-0516-5

[152] Santos MA, Geraldi IO, Garcia AAF, Bortolatto N, Schiavon A, Hungria M. Mapping of QTLs associated with biological nitrogen fixation traits in soybean. Hereditas. 2013;**150**:17-25. DOI: 10.1111/j.1601-5223.2013.02275.x

[153] Yamaguchi-Shinozaki K, Shinozaki K. Transcriptional regulatory networks in cellular responses and tolerance to dehydration and cold stresses. Annual Review of Plant Biology. 2006;**57**:781-803. DOI: 10.1146/annurev.arplant.57.032905.105444

[154] Hu H, Dai M, Yao J, Xiao B, Li X, Zhang Q, et al. Overexpressing a NAM, ATAF, and CUC [NAC] transcription factor enhances drought resistance and salt tolerance in rice. Proceedings of the National Academy of Sciences. 2006;**103**:12987-12992. DOI: 10.1073/pnas.0604882103

[155] Liao Y, Zou H-F, Wei W, Hao Y-J, Tian A-G, Huang J, et al. Soybean GmbZIP44, GmbZIP62 and GmbZIP78 genes function as negative regulator of ABA signaling and confer salt and freezing tolerance in transgenic Arabidopsis. Planta. 2008;**228**:225-240. DOI: 10.1007/s00425-008-0731-3

[156] Zhou QY, Tian AG, Zou HF, Xie ZM, Lei G, Huang J, et al. Soybean WRKY-type transcription factor genes, GmWRKY13, GmWRKY21, and GmWRKY54, confer differential tolerance to abiotic stresses in transgenic *Arabidopsis* plants. Plant Biotechnology Journal. 2008;**6**:486-503. DOI: 10.1111/j.1467-7652.2008.00336.x

[157] Wang N, Zhang W, Qin M, Li S, Qiao M, Liu Z, et al. Drought tolerance conferred in soybean (*Glycine max*. L) by GmMYB84, a novel R2R3-MYB transcription factor. Plant and Cell Physiology. 2017;**58**:1764-1776. DOI: 10.1093/pcp/pcx111

[158] Su L-T, Li J-W, Liu D-Q, Zhai Y, Zhang H-J, Li X-W, et al. A novel MYB transcription factor, GmMYBJ1, from soybean confers drought and cold tolerance in *Arabidopsis thaliana*. Gene. 2014;**538**:46-55. DOI: 10.1016/j.gene.2014.01.024

[159] Li Y, Chen Q, Nan H, Li X, Lu S, Zhao X, et al. Overexpression of GmFDL19 enhances tolerance to drought and salt stresses in soybean. PLoS One. 2017;**12**:e0179554. DOI: 10.1371/journal.pone.0179554

[160] Gao S-Q, Chen M, Xu Z-S, Zhao C-P, Li L, Xu H-J, et al. The soybean GmbZIP1 transcription factor enhances multiple abiotic stress tolerances in transgenic plants. Plant Molecular Biology. 2011;**75**:537-553. DOI: 10.1007/s11103-011-9738-4

[161] Tan DX, Tuong HM, Thuy VTT, Son LV, Mau CH. Cloning and overexpression of GmDREB2 gene from a vietnamese drought-resistant soybean variety. Brazilian Archives of Biology and Technology. 2015;**58**:651-657. DOI: 10.13140/RG.2.1.3642.3126

[162] Mizoi J, Shinozaki K, Yamaguchi-Shinozaki K. AP2/ERF family transcription factors in plant abiotic stress responses. Biochimica et Biophysica Acta Gene Regulatory Mechanisms. 2012;**1819**:86-96. DOI: 10.1016/j.bbagrm.2011.08.004

[163] Zhang G, Chen M, Li L, Xu Z, Chen X, Guo J, et al. Overexpression of the soybean GmERF3 gene, an AP_2/ERF type transcription factor for increased tolerances to salt, drought, and diseases in transgenic tobacco. Journal of Experimental Botany. 2009;**60**:3781-3796. DOI: 10.1093/jxb/erp214

[164] Zhang G, Chen M, Chen X, Xu Z, Li L, Guo J, et al. Isolation and characterization of a novel EAR-motif-containing gene GmERF4 from soybean (*Glycine max* L.). Molecular Biology Reports. 2010;**37**:809-818. DOI: 10.1007/s11033-009-9616-1

[165] Luo X, Bai X, Sun X, Zhu D, Liu B, Ji W, et al. Expression of wild soybean WRKY20 in Arabidopsis enhances drought tolerance and regulates ABA signalling. Journal of Experimental Botany. 2013;**64**:2155-2169. DOI: 10.1093/jxb/ert073

[166] Hao YJ, Wei W, Song QX, Chen HW, Zhang YQ, Wang F, et al. Soybean NAC transcription factors promote abiotic stress tolerance and lateral root formation in transgenic plants. The Plant Journal. 2011;**68**:302-313. DOI: 10.1111/j.1365-313X.2011.04687.x

[167] Chen X, Chen Z, Zhao H, Zhao Y, Cheng B, Xiang Y. Genome-wide analysis of soybean HD-zip gene family and expression profiling under salinity and drought treatments. PLoS One. 2014;**9**:e87156. DOI: 10.1371/journal.pone.0087156

[168] Zhang D, Tong J, Xu Z, Wei P, Xu L, Wan Q, et al. Soybean C_2H_2-type zinc finger protein $GmZFP_3$ with conserved QALGGH motif negatively regulates drought responses in transgenic Arabidopsis. Frontiers in Plant Science. 2016;**7**:325. DOI: 10.3389/fpls.2016.00325

[169] Xie Z-M, Zou H-F, Lei G, Wei W, Zhou Q-Y, Niu C-F, et al. Soybean trihelix transcription factors GmGT-2A and GmGT-2B improve plant tolerance to abiotic stresses in transgenic Arabidopsis. PLoS One. 2009;**4**:e6898. DOI: 10.1371/journal.pone.0006898

[170] Mochida K, Yoshida T, Sakurai T, Yamaguchi-Shinozaki K, Shinozaki K. Tran L-SP. In silico analysis of transcription factor repertoire and prediction of stress responsive transcription factors in soybean. DNA Research. 2009;**16**:3533-3569. DOI: 10.1093/dnares/dsp023

[171] Schmutz J, Cannon SB, Schlueter J, Ma J, Mitros T, Nelson W, et al. Genome sequence of the palaeopolyploid soybean. Nature. 2009;**463**:178-183. DOI: 10.1038/nature08670

[172] Wang F, Chen HW, Li QT, Wei W, Li W, Zhang WK, et al. GmWRKY27 interacts with GmMYB174 to reduce expression of GmNAC29 for stress tolerance in soybean plants. The Plant Journal. 2015;**83**:224-236. DOI: 10.1111/tpj.12879

[173] Tripathi P, Rabara RC, Shen QJ, Rushton PJ. Transcriptomics analyses of soybean leaf and root samples during water-deficit. Genomics Data. 2015;**5**:164-166. DOI: 10.1016/j.gdata.2015.05.036

[174] Jin J, Zhang H, Kong L, Gao G, Luo J. PlantTFDB 3.0: A portal for the functional and evolutionary study of plant transcription factors. Nucleic Acids Research. 2013;**42**: 1182-1187. DOI: 10.1093/nar/gkt1016

[175] Qi Q. Effect of transgenic *DREB3* drought resistant soybean on soil enzyme activity and soil functional microorganism [thesis]. Northeast Agricultural University. 2011

[176] VanToai TT, St Martin SK, Chase K, Boru G, Schnipke V, Schmitthenner AF, et al. Identification of a QTL associated with tolerance of soybean to soil waterlogging. Crop Science. 2001;**41**:1247-1252

[177] Cornelious B, Chen P, Chen Y, De Leon N, Shannon J, Wang D. Identification of QTLs underlying water-logging tolerance in soybean. Molecular Breeding. 2005;**16**:103-112. DOI: 10.1007/s11032-005-5911-2

[178] Githiri S, Watanabe S, Harada K, Takahashi R. QTL analysis of flooding tolerance in soybean at an early vegetative growth stage. Plant Breeding. 2006;**125**:613-618. DOI: 10.1111/j.1439-0523.2006.01291.x

[179] Nguyen V, Vuong T, VanToai T, Lee J, Wu X, Mian M, et al. Mapping of quantitative trait loci associated with resistance to and flooding tolerance in soybean. Crop Science. 2012;**52**:2481-2493. DOI: 10.2135/cropsci2011.09.0466

[180] Sun H, Zhao T, Gai J. Inheritance and QTL mapping of waterlogging tolerance at seedling stage of soybean. Acta Agronomica Sinica. 2010;**36**:590-595. DOI: 10.3724/SP.J.1006.2010.00590

[181] Van Nguyen L, Takahashi R, Githiri SM, Rodriguez TO, Tsutsumi N, Kajihara S, et al. Mapping quantitative trait loci for root development under hypoxia conditions in soybean (*Glycine max* L. Merr.). Theoretical and Applied Genetics. 2017;**130**:743-755. DOI: 10.1007/s00122-016-2847-3

[182] Reyna N, Cornelious B, Shannon J, Sneller C. Evaluation of a QTL for waterlogging tolerance in southern soybean germplasm. Crop Science. 2003;**43**:2077-2082. DOI: 10.1007/s11032-005-5911-2

[183] Cornelious B, Chen P, Hou A, Shi A, Shannon J. Yield potential and waterlogging tolerance of selected near-isogenic lines and recombinant inbred lines from two southern soybean populations. Journal of Crop Improvement. 2006;**16**:97-111. DOI: 10.1300/J411v16n0107

[184] Komatsu S, Yamamoto R, Nanjo Y, Mikami Y, Yunokawa H, Sakata K. A comprehensive analysis of the soybean genes and proteins expressed under flooding stress using transcriptome and proteome techniques. Journal of Proteome Research. 2009;**8**:4766-4778. DOI: 10.1021/pr900460x

[185] Nanjo Y, Maruyama K, Yasue H, Yamaguchi-Shinozaki K, Shinozaki K, Komatsu S. Transcriptional responses to flooding stress in roots including hypocotyl of soybean seedlings. Plant Molecular Biology. 2011;**77**:129-144. DOI: 10.1007/s11103-011-9799-4

[186] Chen W, Yao Q, Patil GB, Agarwal G, Deshmukh RK, Lin L, et al. Identification and comparative analysis of differential gene expression in soybean leaf tissue under drought and flooding stress revealed by RNA-Seq. Frontiers in Plant Science. 2016;**7**:1044. DOI: 10.3389/fpls.2016.01044

[187] Yin X, Hiraga S, Hajika M, Nishimura M, Komatsu S. Transcriptomic analysis reveals the flooding tolerant mechanism in flooding tolerant line and abscisic acid treated soybean. Plant Molecular Biology. 2017;**93**:479-496. DOI: 10.1007/s11103-016-0576-2

[188] Komatsu S, Han C, Nanjo Y, Altaf-Un-Nahar M, Wang K, He D, et al. Label-free quantitative proteomic analysis of abscisic acid effect in early-stage soybean under flooding. Journal of Proteome Research. 2013;**12**:4769-4784. DOI: 10.1021/pr4001898

[189] Oh M, Komatsu S. Characterization of proteins in soybean roots under flooding and drought stresses. Journal of Proteomics. 2015;**114**:161-181. DOI: 10.1016/j.jprot.2014.11.008

[190] Wang X, Oh M, Sakata K, Komatsu S. Gel-free/label-free proteomic analysis of root tip of soybean over time under flooding and drought stresses. Journal of Proteomics. 2016;**130**:42-55. DOI: 10.1016/j.jprot.2015.09.007

[191] Yin X, Komatsu S. Nuclear proteomics reveals the role of protein synthesis and chromatin structure in root tip of soybean during the initial stage of flooding stress. Journal of Proteome Research. 2016;**15**:2283-2298. DOI: 10.1021/acs.jproteome.6b00330

[192] Komatsu S, Sakata K, Nanjo Y. 'Omics' techniques and their use to identify how soybean responds to flooding. Journal of Analytical Science and Technology. 2015;**6**:9. DOI: 10.1186/s40543-015-0052-7

[193] Komatsu S, Nanjo Y, Nishimura M. Proteomic analysis of the flooding tolerance mechanism in mutant soybean. Journal of Proteomics. 2013;**79**:231-250. DOI: 10.1016/j.jprot.2012.12.023

[194] Wang Z, Li P, Yang Y, Chi Y, Fan B, Chen Z. Expression and functional analysis of a novel Group of Legume-Specific WRKY and Exo70 protein variants from soybean. Scientific Reports. 2016;**6**:32090. DOI: 10.1038/srep32090

[195] Yin X, Nishimura M, Hajika M, Komatsu S. Quantitative proteomics reveals the flooding-tolerance mechanism in mutant and abscisic acid-treated soybean. Journal of Proteome Research. 2016;**15**:2008-2025. DOI: 10.1021/acs.jproteome.6b00196

[196] Chang R, Qiu L. Evaluation and utilization of soybean germplasm in China. In: Lam HM, Chang R, Shao G, Liu Z, editors. Research on Tolerance to Stresses in Chinese Soybean. Beijing: China Agricultural Press; 2009

[197] Xu Z, Chang R, Qiu L, Sun J, Li X, editors. Evaluation of soybean germplasm in China. In: Proceedings of the World Soybean Research Conference VI, Chicago; August 1999. pp. 4-7

[198] Lam H-M, Xu X, Liu X, Chen W, Yang G, Wong F-L, et al. Resequencing of 31 wild and cultivated soybean genomes identifies patterns of genetic diversity and selection. Nature Genetics. 2010;**42**:1053-1059. DOI: 10.1038/ng.715

[199] Christou P, McCabe DE, Swain WF. Stable transformation of soybean callus by DNA-coated gold particles. Plant Physiology. 1988;**87**:671-674

[200] Hinchee MA, Connor-Ward DV, Newell CA, McDonnell RE, Sato SJ, Gasser CS, et al. Production of transgenic soybean plants using agrobacterium-mediated DNA transfer. Biotechnology. 1988;**6**:915-922. DOI: 10.1038/nbt0888-915

[201] Dang W, Z-m W. An optimized agrobacterium-mediated transformation for soybean for expression of binary insect resistance genes. Plant Science. 2007;**173**:381-389. DOI: 10.1016/j.plantsci.2007.06.010

[202] Paz MM, Shou H, Guo Z, Zhang Z, Banerjee AK, Wang K. Assessment of conditions affecting agrobacterium-mediated soybean transformation using the cotyledonary node explant. Euphytica. 2004;**136**:167-179. DOI: 10.1007/s00299-005-0113-2

[203] Farooq M, Wahid A, Kobayashi N, Fujita D, Basra S. Plant drought stress: Effects, mechanisms and management. Agronomy for Sustainable Development. 2009;**29**:185-212. DOI: 10.1051/agro:2008021

[204] Zhang M, Duan L, Zhai Z, Li J, Tian X, Wang B, et al., editors. Effects of plant growth regulators on water deficit-induced yield loss in soybean. In: Proceedings of the 4th International Crop Science Congress, Brisbane, Australia. September 26, 2004. pp. 252-256

[205] Barta R, Broner I, Schneekloth J, Waskom R. Colorado high plains irrigation practices guide: Water saving options for irrigators in Eastern Colorado. Colorado Water Resources Research Institute Special Report No 14. 2004

[206] Guo ZL, Sun CQ, Liang N. Impacts of plastic mulching on water saving and yield increasing of dry land spring soybean and its density effect. Chinese Journal of Eco-Agriculture. 2007;**1**:053

[207] Zurweller BA. Nitrogen Fertilizer Management of Temporarily Waterlogged Soils to Improve Corn Production and Reduce Environmental Nitrogen Loss. Columbia: University of Missouri; 2014

[208] Wang M, Zheng Q, Shen Q, Guo S. The critical role of potassium in plant stress response. International Journal of Molecular Sciences. 2013;**14**:7370-7390. DOI: 10.3390/ijms14047370

[209] Martinelle K, Häggström L. Mechanisms of ammonia and ammonium ion toxicity i3n animal cells: Transport across cell membranes. Journal of Biotechnology. 1993;**30**:339-350. DOI: 10.1016/0168-1656[93]90148-G

[210] Ashraf MA, Ahmad MSA, Ashraf M, Al-Qurainy F, Ashraf MY. Alleviation of waterlogging stress in upland cotton [*Gossypium hirsutum* L.] by exogenous application of potassium in soil and as a foliar spray. Crop and Pasture Science. 2011;**62**:25-38. DOI: 10.1071/CP09225

[211] Liu G, Li Y, Migliaccio K, Olczyk T, Alva A. Oxygen amendment on growth and nitrogen use efficiency of flooded Italian basil. International Journal of Vegetable Science. 2013;**19**:217-227. DOI: 10.1080/19315260.2012.713451

[212] Li G, Meng X, Wang R, Mao G, Han L, Liu Y, et al. Dual-level regulation of ACC synthase activity by MPK3/MPK6 cascade and its downstream WRKY transcription factor during ethylene induction in Arabidopsis. PLOS Genetics. 2012;**8**:e1002767. DOI: 10.1371/journal.pgen.1002767

[213] Else MA, Jackson MB. Transport of 1-aminocyclopropane-1-carboxylic acid [ACC] in the transpiration stream of tomato (*Lycopersicon esculentum*) in relation to foliar ethylene production and petiole epinasty. Functional Plant Biology. 1998;**25**:453-458. DOI: 10.1071/PP97105

[214] Grichko VP, Glick BR. Amelioration of flooding stress by ACC deaminase-containing-plant growth-promoting bacteria. Plant Physiology and Biochemistry. 2001;**39**:11-17. DOI: 10.1016/S0981-9428[00]01212-2

[215] Barnawal D, Bharti N, Maji D, Chanotiya CS, Kalra A. 1-Aminocyclopropane-1-carboxylic acid (ACC) deaminase-containing rhizobacteria protect *Ocimum sanctum* plants during waterlogging stress via reduced ethylene generation. Plant Physiology and Biochemistry. 2012;**58**:227-235. DOI: 10.1016/j.plaphy.2012.07.008

[216] Li J, McConkey BJ, Cheng Z, Guo S, Glick BR. Identification of plant growth-promoting bacteria-responsive proteins in cucumber roots under hypoxic stress using a proteomic approach. Journal of Proteomics. 2013;**84**:119-131. DOI: 10.1016/j.jprot.2013.03.011

Chapter 4

Sugar Beet Tolerance to Drought: Physiological and Molecular Aspects

Marina Putnik-Delić, Ivana Maksimović,
Nevena Nagl and Branislava Lalić

Additional information is available at the end of the chapter

http://dx.doi.org/10.5772/intechopen.72253

Abstract

Drought often reduces sugar beet yield in the Balkan agroecological region. Climate forecasts indicate that this negative trend of drought periods will continue. Tolerance to drought is a complex trait, which comprises involvement of both physiological and molecular mechanisms in plants. This research was conducted on 11 sugar beet genotypes, which showed different tolerance to drought in the field. Experiment had three parts: water deficiency caused by cessation of watering conducted in the greenhouse, water deficiency imposed by different concentrations of polyethylene glycol on plants grown in tissue culture, and analysis of alterations in gene expression under drought. Plants exposed to stress in greenhouse had on average three leaves less, 4% lower water content, and seven-fold higher proline content. Classification of genotypes with respect to the level of tolerance to water deficiency on the basis of concentration of free proline, assessed in the experiment *in vitro*, corresponded to the result of the observation test in the field. Changes in the expression of candidate genes under drought suggest that one of them might be used for further development as a DNA-based marker. These results can be applied in sugar beet breeding aimed at increasing tolerance to water deficiency.

Keywords: water deficiency, *Beta vulgaris*, drought tolerance, polyethylene glycol, chloroplast pigments, chlorophyll fluorescence, free proline, green house, tissue culture, candidate genes

1. Introduction

1.1. Amount and distribution of precipitation required for sugar beet development

Required amount of precipitation for successful production of sugar beet is 600 mm per year [1]. Furthermore, during the winter period, sugar beet requires around 230 mm and during the period of vegetation (from April to October) approximately 370 mm of precipitate. However, based on perennial average yield data, sugar beet production may achieve high outcome even in the presence of lower (500 mm per year) or higher (1000 mm per year) amount of rain. Water requirement of plant, during the period of vegetation, depends on precipitation. The water loss due to evaporation is most intensive from June to August when the temperatures are high and the air is dry. The average potential evapotranspiration (ET) for period of 30 years in case of sugar beet is 576 mm, but it may vary between 528 and 625 mm due to weather conditions. Approximately 10–20% of total water requirement of sugar beet is fulfilled from the soil water reserves and the rest is obtained by precipitation and irrigation. The amount of water lost by transpiration is 392 mm in average, and it varies from 198 mm during dry years to 542 mm during rainy years. The average precipitation during vegetation (April–September) is 359 mm and it varies from 138 to 521 mm in certain years [2].

Having in mind the above-mentioned facts, amount and distribution of precipitation, in combination with the light and amount of heat, mostly determine quality and yield of sugar beet. On the territory of Serbia, it is common that the lack of soil water, typical for summer months, sometimes occurs during moderately rained years. Lack of soil moisture outcomes 100–200 mm per year, but rarely exceeds 300 mm per year. Currently, less than 1% of irrigation-suitable agricultural land in Serbia is intensively irrigated.

Climate of Serbia is continental or moderate continental. The most important sugar beet production area is Vojvodina region situated in the north of the country. Climate of Vojvodina is moderated continental, determined by the presence of Alps on western border of Pannonian basin, Carpathian Mountains, the Dinarides, and the Balkan Mountains [3]. Precipitation regime is continental, typical for Danube region, with precipitation maximum in summer (June) and minimum in winter. According to the Köppen classification [4], for the period of 1961–1990, dominant climate type in Vojvodina is *Cfwbx″* [*C* = mild temperate climate; *f* = significant precipitation during all seasons; *w* = dry winters; *b* = warmest month averaging below 22°C (but with at least 4 months averaging above 10°C) and *x″* = second precipitation maximum occurs in autumn] [5].

Brief analysis of current and expected precipitation distribution during winter, spring, and sugar beet growing season in Vojvodina is made using the data from two meteorological stations located in southern and northwestern part of the Vojvodina region, Novi Sad (Rimski Sancevi) and Sombor, respectively. Climatological data for 1971–2000 refers to the climatological periods derived from the database of the Republic Hydrometeorological Service of Serbia (RHMSS). Future climatic conditions were obtained from the Eta Belgrade University (EBU)—Princeton Ocean Model (POM) model for the A1B scenario for 2001–2030 and A2 for 2071–2100 integration periods [6]. Obtained results lead to expected shift in climate types from *Cfwbx* to "*Cfwax*" in the prevailing part of the country indicating temperature of the warmest month above 22°C (letter *a* in the Köppen formula) [5].

Overview of the average precipitation for the selected past climatological period indicates that during winter time of 1971–2000 reference period, the amount of precipitation is twice less than optimum ones, while growing period of precipitation was slightly below optimal values.

According to climate model simulations for 2001–2030 integration periods, expected average annual precipitation during first decades of the twentieth century, at selected locations, will not vary significantly in relation to the 1971–2000 precipitation records (**Table 1**). Inspection of the precipitation amounts for 2001–2014 period (**Table 2**) witnesses in favor to this expectation, with 699.8 mm in Novi Sad and 668.0 mm in Sombor in comparison with the expected 2001–2030 average (**Table 1**). However, it is important to notice significant variability of precipitation in this period which is in accordance with climate simulations for 2001–2030 [3]. In regards to winter and spring precipitations, for all integration periods, climate model simulates slightly higher average precipitation in comparison to reference climatology. Less optimistic is the expectation that growing period precipitation supposed to decrease towards end of the century, with particularly vulnerable summer period and increasing variability.

1.2. The impact of water deficiency on sugar beet production

Water shortage during vegetation is a frequent and a significant issue in agricultural production. Possible solution to this problem is selection of genotypes, which do not show decreased yield under economically acceptable level, in the presence of water shortage. Great challenge in the process of genotype selection is to choose the convenient plant idiotype for the present agroecological conditions. Water deficiency has complex impact on plant physiology. First indicators of water deficiency in plants are the loss of turgor pressure and stomatal closure [7]. Photosynthesis is also highly dependable on the plant's water supply. Many studies showed that disruption of water flow causes decrease in water content in assimilation tissue, which leads to photosynthetic depression [8]. Based on this, soil moisture, as well as relative air humidity, determines photosynthetic intensity. A decrease in chloroplast size, an increase

Climatol. period	Annual	Winter (DJF)		Spring (MAM)		Growing season	
	Precipitation (mm)	Precipitation (mm)	Variability coeff. (%)	Precipitation (mm)	Variability coeff. (%)	Precipitation (mm)	Variability coeff. (%)
	Novi Sad (Rimski Sancevi)						
1971–2000	604.1	108.1	46.2	146.6	33.3	359.2	28.8
2001–2030	641.8	131.3	56.1	159.7	34.7	369.2	26.1
2071–2100	560.5	131.0	54.5	147.4	37.0	282.2	32.0
	Sombor						
1971–2000	580.3	107.6	41.9	133.3	29.6	339.4	22.7
2001–2030	629.4	127.3	56.7	144.6	37.2	356.5	29.0
2071–2100	565.8	127.2	53.6	148.1	41.3	277.8	31.9

Table 1. Past (1971–2000) and future (2001–2030 and 2071–2100) climate precipitation data for Novi Sad and Sombor locations in Serbia.

Year	Novi Sad (Rimski Sancevi)	Sombor
2000	252	231
2001	929	749
2002	412	448
2003	491	434
2004	797	816
2005	726	753
2006	640	585
2007	754	683
2008	539	598
2009	617	615
2010	1035	994
2011	382	401
2012	480	446
2013	723	692
2014	989	932
Average	679.8	653.3

Table 2. Annual amount of precipitation for 2001–2014 in Novi Sad (Rimski Sancevi) and Sombor locations.

in stomatal density, and disruption of thylakoid membrane structure were reported as consequences of water deficit [9]. Besides decrease in tissue water content, water shortage may cause synthesis of specific compounds in the roots, during the early growth phase. According to this, roots are very significant sensors of soil changes (not only in terms of water, but also texture changes), which alert the aboveground tissues by "chemical drought signals" which are transported to leaves. These signals mostly refer to plant hormones such as abscisic acid (ABA) [10].

1.3. Sugar beet tolerance to water deficiency

Adaptation of plant metabolism on stress conditions is species specific and was the subject of numerous studies [11]. Plants more tolerant to drought have longer root system with bigger absorptive area, better developed photosynthetic parenchyma, thicker cuticle, smaller leaf area (LA) and number of stomata per leaf area, and higher density of conductive elements [12]. They also possess highly expandable protoplasm, higher content of bound water and osmolytes, enhanced accumulation of ABA, free proline, and alanine. The following indicators point out to higher phenotypic tolerance of sugar beet to water shortage: more shiny leaves, higher turgor pressure of petiole, and more sensitive leaves to expansion [12]. Even though there is genotypic variability with respect to response to drought in sugar beet (i.e., [13]), structural and morphological mechanisms still remain unclear.

Stress occurrence during early stages of growth and development may adversely affect sugar beet root growth, which may result in yield loss by 46% [14]. In addition, later stress occurrence may cause decreased leaf area and also number of leaves and by that, the efficiency in light usage becomes decreased [15]. Water deficiency significantly increases concentrations of potassium and sodium, which disturb sugar extraction from roots. Plant response to water stress can partially be explained by disorders in mineral nutrition. Water deficiency actually may retard or even stop ion assimilation, which results in perturbation in ion ratios in specific tissues. This trend is manifested through ion deficiency symptoms in plants. The adverse effect of water stress in later phenophases is less pronounced, since plants already developed root system and canopy which completely covers the soil. Well-developed root system increases efficiency in water extraction and usage, which results in higher tolerance to water deficiency [16]. However, first signs of water stress are usually seen on leaves. Minor drop in leaf water potential may cause significant decrease of total leaf area, and the low water potential enhances emergence of new leaves and accelerates senescence of old leaves. Drought stress results in stomatal closure, limits the transpiration which increases leaf temperature [15]. Both, lower stomatal density and heat stress decrease photosynthetic outcome [17]. Sugar beet leaves have higher number of smaller stomata on their abaxial side. Higher density and smaller size of stomata is a form of adaptation to drought, because it allows plants to be more efficient in regulation of water transport and transpiration [18]. Varieties more efficient in tolerating lack of water are proven to have decreased stomatal density (70–150 stomata/mm^2) [19]. During drought, when negative turgor pressure in guard cells generates, small epidermal cells with tightened cell walls increase plant resistance towards water stress [20]. Response of sugar beet genotypes to drought may also be affected by percentage of adaxial and abaxial epidermis and palisade tissue thickness [21].

1.4. Chemical response of sugar beet to drought stress

Plants also osmotically adapt to drought [22]. Exposure to water deficiency results in accumulation of osmolytes, such as betaine, proline, and fructans. These substances often accumulate in the form of compatible solutes in plants (compounds which do not take part in chemical reactions in plants, but affect cell water potential), which generate expression of genes encoding relevant enzymes. Osmolyte production, as well as change in osmotic pressure, may increase sugar beet tolerance to abiotic stress. Proline and glycine betaine help in the preservation of cell [23], which makes them suitable for further investigation with purpose of increase stress tolerance of many species including sugar beet [24, 25]. They are not only involved in maintenance of cell turgor and osmotic balance but also in protection of cell structure from stress [26]. However, it still remains unclear whether the plants, which accumulate osmolytes, better tolerate lack of water or not [27].

1.5. Proline accumulation

Free proline is a key metabolite which accumulates in sugar beet exposed to drought [28]. Change of the free proline concentrations in tissues is an indicator of other kinds of stress, such as temperature, environmental pollution, and misbalanced nutrition. The same factors may affect glucose accumulation and yield. In some cases, stress conditions may increase sugar beet root quality and potential of recovery if plants were not highly damaged by water deficiency [29].

Higher nitrogen supply increases proline content and may also increase leaf area index (LAI) and drought stress impact. Positive and significant correlation among proline and glucose content in sugar beet root indicates the relationship between the response to stress, carbohydrates, and proline and glucose accumulation ratio. This is supported by the effect of treatment with di-1-p-mentene (anti-transpirant) and DMDP (2,5-dihydroxymetil-3,4-dihydroxypyrolidine, glycosidase inhibitor), which decreased proline content in roots of irrigated sugar beet [29]. Presence of compounds such as proline and glucose adversely affect sugar crystallization and lead to the formation of colored components, thus reducing industrial quality of beet roots [30].

Proline accumulated in sugar beet root, as a nitrogen compound, reduces the quality of roots. Both, the stress and an excess of nitrogen lead to the mobilization of accumulated carbohydrates, which are the source of energy essential for adaptation to the stress conditions. Moreover, chemicals containing nitrogen (e.g., proline) reduce the yield of sucrose and the quality of the roots [29]. The importance of the accumulation of proline in osmotic adjustment is still debatable and varies from species to species [31]. The highest proline accumulation was observed at the end of beet root growth [29]. Correlation between drought and proline content suggests, however, that alteration in proline concentration is useful stress indicator in sugar beet [28]. Proline may act as a signal molecule which alters mitochondrial function, affects cell division and gene expression. This role of proline may be very significant for plant recovery when favorable conditions are regained [32].

1.6. The use of plant biotechnology to increase tolerance to water deficiency

Basic need for sustainable food production directed research programs towards improving traits of crops despite the size and complexity of their genome [33]. Plant biotechnology is a process in which the use of molecular and cytological techniques help to increase the productivity of the plants, to improve the quality of plant products, to prevent the damage caused under the influence of various biotic and abiotic stresses. Plant breeding reliving on the employment of molecular markers [Marker Assisted Selection (MAS)] is one of the promising techniques to improve crop resilience. A prerequisite for the success of MAS is defining the genes which regulate traits of interest and to test relationships between potential markers and those traits. Only when this link is defined, i.e., when the marker is physically located in the vicinity of or even within the gene of interest, it is possible to use it efficiently in breeding [34].

In sugar beet, development of breeding programs aimed to increase drought tolerance is further complicated by the fact that several types of abiotic stresses often occur at the same time during the growing season, and approach which involves a manipulation of a group of genes for tolerance to drought seems necessary to solve this complex problem [35].

In an era of rapid progress in the identification and characterization of complete segments of plant genome, proteins, transcripts, metabolites, as well as their interactions in a biological system, new discoveries will lead to better understanding and possibly to manipulation of physiological responses to water deficit [36]. Evaluation of the relative contribution of genes conferring tolerance to the dehydration and elimination of those which do not affect the tolerance to stress is a major challenge.

Although the yield is the basic goal of the breeders, it is very difficult to accurately predict the possibility of water utilization and identify candidate genes for further cloning [37]. Several studies have identified quantitative trait loci (QTLs) associated with a specific component of the response to drought. Although the development of molecular markers and genome sequencing should expedite positional cloning [38], genome areas associated with individual QTLs are still very large and usually not suitable for testing in the breeding program. With the rapid development of genomic technology and the suitable statistical methods, there is an increased interest in the use of mapping strategies for the identification of genes encoding quantitative traits which have agricultural or evolutionary significance [11]. Another major challenge is how to apply knowledge to improve crop tolerance to stress conditions. There is a problem between high yield and tolerance to stress since very often genotypes with higher stress tolerance have lower yield under optimal conditions. One of the strategies for sugar beet phenotyping was proposed by Ries et al. [39].

On the cellular level plant adaptation to stress includes regulation of the beginning of protein synthesis (e.g., H^+ pumps and Na^+/H^+ antiporter), an increase in antioxidant level, transient increase of the concentrations of ABA, the reduction of the energy consumption ways, as well as accumulation of the solution, and protective protein [40]. All of these changes at the cellular level are of great importance for the maintenance of homeostasis after ion imbalance caused by abiotic stress [26]. The deficit of water causes the synthesis and accumulation of ABA in plant cells and the genes corresponding to this has been defined. Most of these genes contain conserved cis-activating promoter elements, called Abre (ABA-responsive element, PyACGTGG/TC) [41]. Great progress to clarify the response of plants to abiotic stress has been made in the last decade [11].

In order to achieve a combination of high yield and tolerance to stress in one variety, it is necessary to establish a connection of development of individual characteristics and mutual reactions, which can be achieved only through co-operation among molecular biologists, physiologists, and breeders [11, 42]. It is necessary to assess the relationship between different morphological, anatomical, physiological, and biochemical traits of sugar beet tissues in different phases of their growth and development during different periods of water shortage, in order to categorize genotypes with respect to their tolerance to drought which was in the focus of our previous [21] and present study.

2. Material and methods

2.1. Plant material

The study involved 11 genotypes (marked from 1 to 11) of sugar beet (*Beta vulgaris* ssp. *vulgaris*, L.) differing in levels of drought tolerance, according to observation test conducted in the field. According to this test, genotypes were divided into three groups: (1) sensitive genotypes: 2, 5, 6, and 8; (2) moderately tolerant: 3, 7, 9, and 11; and (3) tolerant: 1, 4, and 10.

Experiment was conducted in three stages:

1. Under semi-controlled conditions in greenhouse.
2. In in vitro conditions of tissue culture.
3. Gene expression analyses of water regime responsible genes in leaves (plants from the greenhouse experiment).

2.1.1. Experiment under semi-controlled conditions in greenhouse

Sugar beet seeds were sown in growth substrate Potgrond H (Klasmann), mixed with river sand (17.5:1) in plastic pots (31 × 37 × 13 cm). A single pot contained 12 plants. During 90-day period, soil moisture was kept at 80% field capacity. Plant watering was conducted on the basis of evapotranspiration. When the plants were at the 6–12 leaves stage, they were exposed to water deficit by cessation of watering, while control plants were watered. Five days later, molecular and physiological analyses were done.

After drying plant material on 105–130°C to its constant mass, % of dry matter was determined. Activity of photosynthetic apparatus was assessed by monitoring of $F_{0(initial)}$, $F_{m(maximal)}$, $F_{v(variable)}$, F_v/F_m, and $t_{1/2}$ using plant stress meter (PSM, BioMonitor S.C.I. AB). Free proline concentration was measured in the both *in vitro* and *in vivo* conditions [43]. Concentration of chloroplast pigments was determined spectrophotometrically [44, 45]. Leaf area (LA) was measured by automatic leaf area meter LI-3000 (LI-COR, USA).

2.1.2. Experiment in tissue culture

In this experiment, MS basic substrate was used [46] with 0.3 mg/l BA (benzyldenine) and 0.01 mg/l GA_3 (gibberellic acid). In order to obtain sufficient number of axillary shoots (64), equal in size, subcultivation was done every 3 weeks. Lack of water was caused by addition of polyethylene glycol to the substrate. Obtained shoots were set on a substrate for micropropagation with 0, 3, and 5% of polyethylene glycol (PEG 6000, Duchefa, Netherlands). Plants were cultivated on this substrate for 4 weeks and afterwards fresh weight of shoots, as well as dry matter and free proline content were determined. The temperature during the experiment in air conditioning chamber was 21–23°C, with a photoperiod of 16 h of light and 8 h of dark.

2.1.3. Gene expression analyses of water regime responsible genes in leaves (plants grew in the first experiment)

The changes in gene expression were analyzed in the leaves of the sugar beet plants grown in the greenhouse experiment. Candidate genes were selected from the previous studies [47–50]. For 13 candidate genes which are, considered to be, involved in osmotic and salt stress responses, primers were constructed and used to screen for polymorphisms at the DNA and gene expression levels. Ten selected candidate genes were homologous probes (BI543470, BI096135, AW697770, BI543640, BG932913, BI096146, BQ060651, BF011094, BI096078, and BF011254), and heterologous probes from maize (X15290), alfalfa (BI543243), and carrot (BI073246). Samples for DNA/RNA analysis (leaves) were taken 5 days after the last watering (experiment 1) and used for DNA/mRNA extractions. mRNA was used to synthesize cDNA, and this cDNA was template in further PCR reactions [42].

2.2. Statistical analyses

Statistical analyses of data were performed by different statistical methods. ANOVA was applied, to photosynthetic pigments (MCMCglmm Methods, [51]), using Package R (http://www.jstatsoft.org/v33/i02/). Logarithmic and Jonson's transformations (Minitab) were performed for parameters with large data variability, in order to normalize their distribution. Confidence intervals for fitted mean responses were calculated as quantiles of simulated distributions of the expected response values. Analyses were done with the R environment [52] and the contributed packages lme4 [53] and ggplot2 [54].

3. Results and discussion

As previously indicated (**Tables 1** and **2**), climatic conditions in our region suggest the need for research, which has the potential to enhance selection of genotypes more tolerant to drought.

3.1. Experiment under semi-controlled conditions in greenhouse

3.1.1. Sugar beet genotype classification based on physiological tests in semi-controlled conditions

Sugar beet genotypes in semi-controlled conditions showed different reactions to 5-day water deficiency. As expected, decline in turgor was observed in all genotypes. Number of leaves was significantly different between treatments and respective controls. Concentrations of photosynthetic pigments and leaf area varied between genotypes and standard normal distribution was not observed here. Therefore, the data were subjected to Johnson's data transformation which proved to be very effective [55]. This procedure allowed assessing differences in concentrations of photosynthetic pigments between different genotypes (**Figure 1**).

Secession in water supply caused water loss from plant tissues within both sensitive and tolerant genotypes. Due to this fact, sugar beet genotypes may be divided on the basis of tested parameters and following treatments (**Figure 2**).

The results obtained in semi-controlled conditions (experiment 1) were compared to previous field observations (**Figure 3**). Proline concentration increased in all genotypes after exposure to water deficit as well as % of DM (except for genotypes 9 and 11). Changes within treatments with respect to control, referring to dry weight were less pronounced than changes referring to % of DM and RWC of root, stem, and leaf. Plants subjected to stress conditions had in average three leaves less, 4% higher % of DM, and seven times higher proline content.

The relationships between two effects on measured traits were assessed by mixed model (**Figure 4**). Crossed pink lines in diagrams represent average impact on genotypes in control

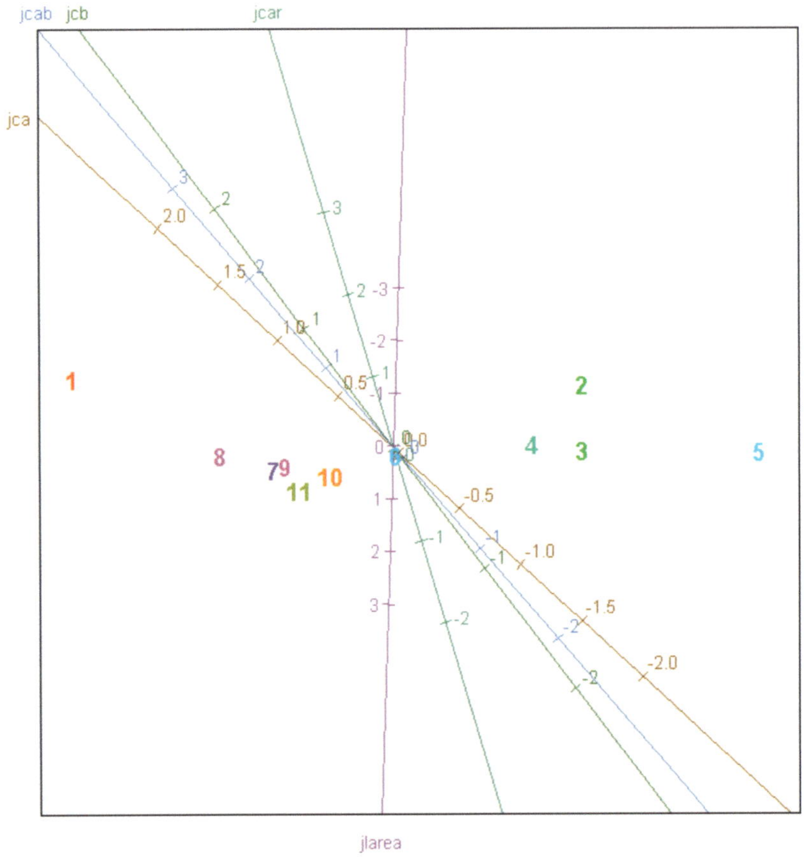

Figure 1. Genotype separation on the basis of pigment concentration and leaf area for variables normalized according to Johnson's data transformation (jlarea—leaf area; jcar—carotenoids; jca—chlorophyll a; jcb—chlorophyll b; jcab—chlorophyll a + b).

(x axis) and stress effect (y axis). There is a nearly perfect negative correlation between the unstressed value and the response to stress for root DM and a similar, but weaker one, for leaf number. Genotypes showing positive scores for the slope effect (y axis) are less affected than the average by (more tolerant to) water stress for the involved trait, and vice-versa. Genotypes showing positive scores for both effects are both higher scoring in absence of stress and less affected than the average by (more tolerant to) stress for the involved trait, and vice-versa.

Conventionally, results of chlorophyll fluorescence indicate a high sensitivity to influence of ecological factors. Therefore, it is often used as an indicator of functioning of photosystem II.

According to F_v/F_m, sugar beet genotypes were compared on the basis of photosynthetic characteristics. Water deficit did not cause significant variations in fluorescence indicators (**Figure 5**).

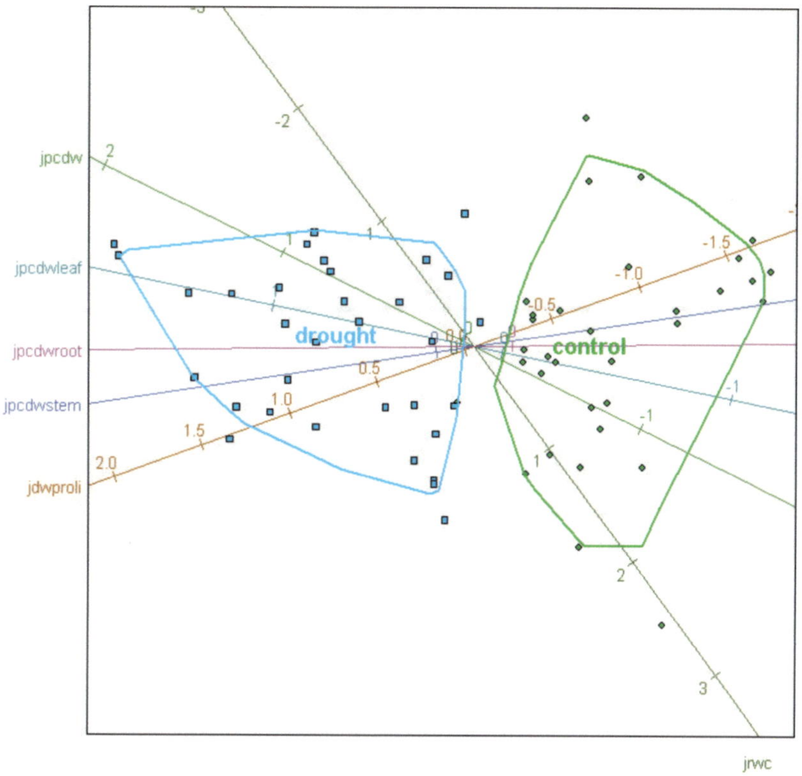

Figure 2. The separation of the sugar beet genotypes based on experiments in greenhouse with a highlighting treatment (control, drought) for a variable normalized by Johnson's transformation (jrwc—relative water content; jpcdw—dry weight; jdwproli—free proline; jpcdwleaf—leaf dry matter; jpcdwstem—stem dry matter; jpcdwroot—root dry matter).

Effects of drought were observed in case of F_v and F_m, but not for F_v/F_m ratio, where the largest differences between genotypes were obtained. In addition, overlap of intervals of interaction between stress and genotype indicates stress, which caused differences, similar for all genotypes. The influence of water deficiency on fluorescence may be related to plant tolerance towards water deficit in field conditions (**Figure 5**).

Plant development may be inhibited in different ways in field conditions. It may be affected by interactions among drought and other ecological stresses, precipitation, and temperature availability as well as interactions with different micro-organisms [36]. On the contrary, semi-controlled conditions may only eliminate interference of other factors with plant development. Therefore, it is necessary to compare results obtained in the greenhouse with those obtained in the field.

3.2. Experiment in tissue culture (*in vitro*)

Increased PEG concentration decreased growth of axillary buds with respect to control (**Figure 6**).

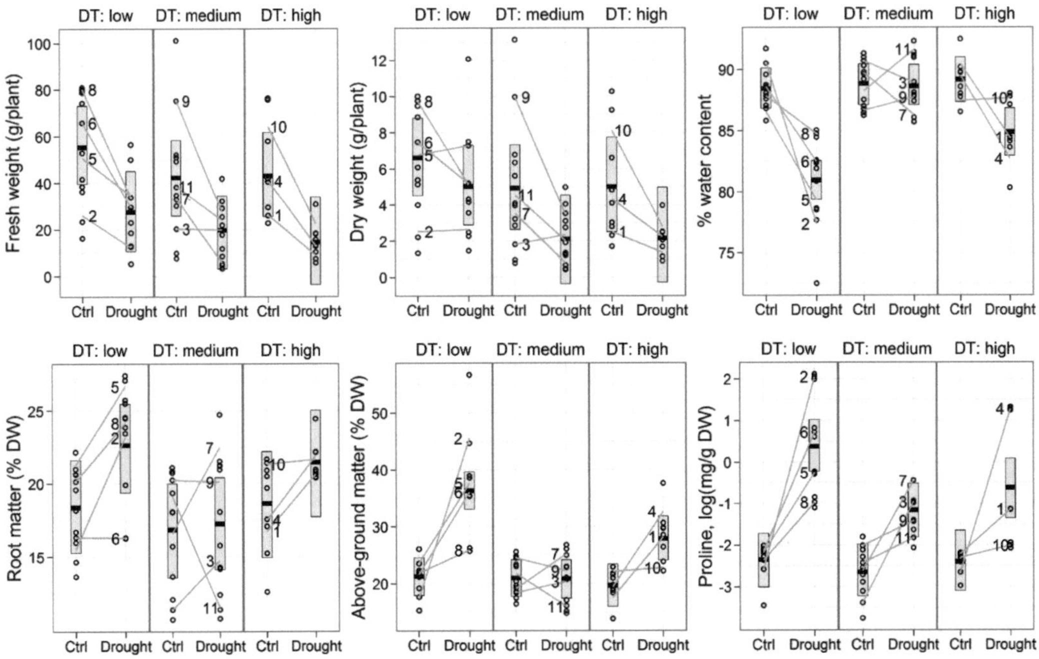

Figure 3. Effects of drought stress on growth traits and proline production of greenhouse grown plants of sugar beet genotypes (1–11) from three classes of visually field-assessed drought tolerance (DT). Observed values of three replicates (circles, 10 plants each), average genotype positions (numbered gray lines), and class means with 95% confidence intervals (crossbars). The drought stress was induced by suspension of watering to test plots after 3 months of culture and observations were made after 5 more days [28].

Number of axillary shoots may be indicator of the influence of different PEG concentrations, which cause water deficit, on micropropagation potential of genotypes. Average number of axillary shoots of 11 subjected genotypes showed 2.2 times decreased number of shoots in the presence of 3% PEG and 2.7 times in the presence of 5% of PEG.

The degree of tolerance to drought observed in the field corresponded to tolerance recorded in the experiments performed in the greenhouse and in tissue culture (**Figure 6**). The most prominent criterion for estimation of genotype tolerance to drought was found to be concentration of free proline [28]. Proline concentration was significantly increased in leaves exposed to drought and axillary buds and it was positively correlated with PEG concentration, which is in accordance with the results of other researches [56].

PEG treatment decreased total dry weight and number of axillary shoots by more than twice, while presence of 3% PEG in the substrate increased total fresh weight. Furthermore, PEG caused decrease in water content in tissues and decreased number of buds, but increased bud weight and % of DM. The highest values were recorded in control (0% PEG) for total fresh weight, in the presence of 3% PEG for proline concentration and fresh weight of axillary buds and in presence of 5% PEG for % of DM. Fresh weight of plants grown in presence of 3 and 5% PEG decreased (**Figure 6**). Average dry weight of the plants was the highest in the presence of 3% PEG. However, in the presence of 5% PEG, it was almost in line with the control. Higher

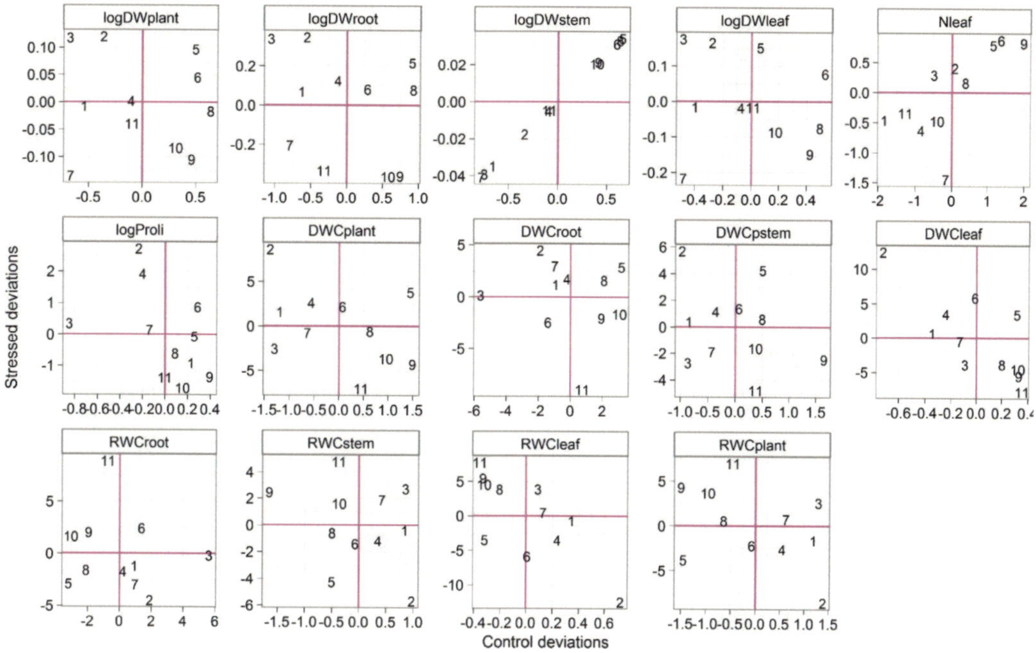

Figure 4. Genotype effects from mixed model analyses for traits of greenhouse experiment (deviations for values in unstressed condition on the x axis, deviations for stress effects on the y axis. Genotypes are identified by the numbers).

variability in dry weight was recorded in the group of drought sensitive group (according to field observations), but the same trend as in the other two groups of genotypes remained. Tissue water content linearly decreased following the increase in PEG concentration, the average drop in presence of 5% PEG was 6%, and was followed by the low average difference among groups of different tolerance and higher difference among genotypes of one group (**Figure 6**).

Proline accumulation under stress conditions increased under treatments in both experiments. In tissue culture, it was 6 times increased and in greenhouse 16 times with respect to corresponding controls.

If taking into account the genotypes tolerance in the field, in relation to the parameters obtained from the analysis of plants in tissue culture and in experiment in the greenhouse, dry matter, in relation to the water content and the concentration of proline is not significantly different among groups of the tolerance (**Figure 7**).

Recorded differences between genotypes show that there are two approaches for the separation of sugar beet genotypes in relation to response to water stress, which cannot substitute each other. On one hand, proline content in plants grown in tissue culture enabled to match their grouping with respect to observations in the field. On the other hand, experiment in greenhouse was less efficient in that sense (**Figure 3**). The main cause of this may be the fact that stress in the field was not continuous as it was in the greenhouse.

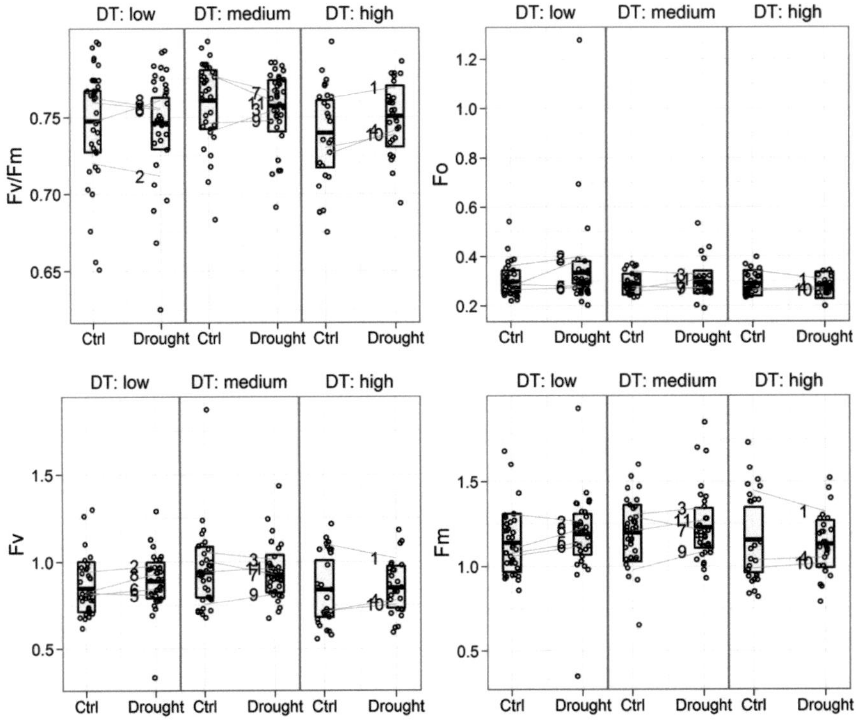

Figure 5. Maximal (F_m) and variable (F_v) chlorophyll fluorescence and their ratio (F_v/F_m) in sugar beet genotypes grouped according to their field-assessed drought tolerance (ctrl—control; drought; DT—drought tolerance).

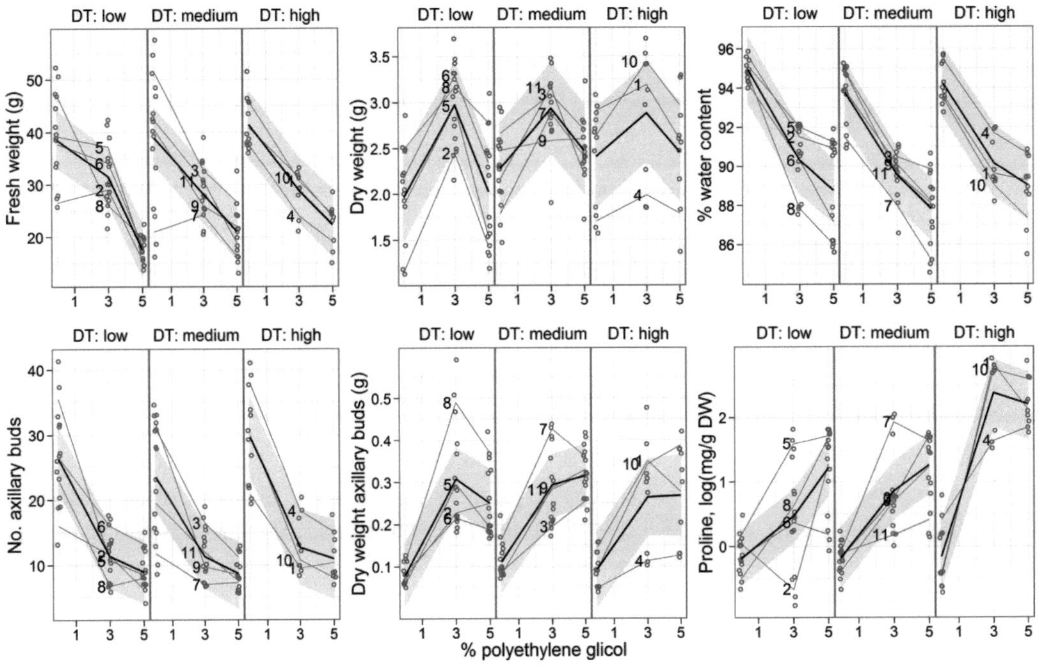

Figure 6. PEG effect on growth traits and free proline concentration of plants cultivated in tissue culture [28].

http://dx.doi.org/10.5772/intechopen.72253

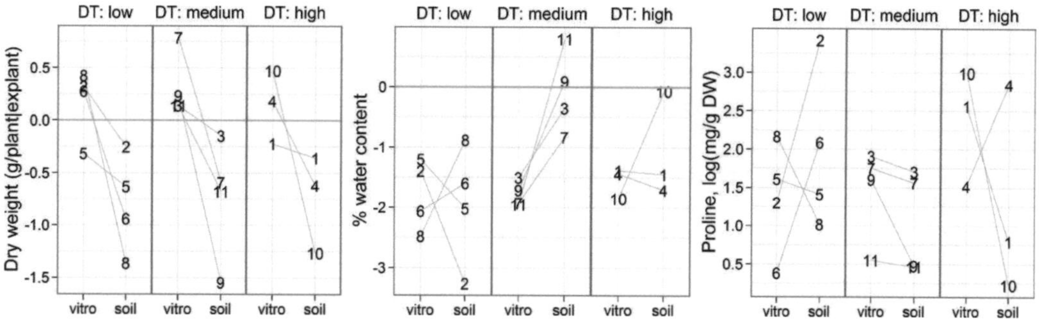

Figure 7. Water deficit effect on dry weight, water content, and free proline concentration in greenhouse and in tissue culture experiment [28].

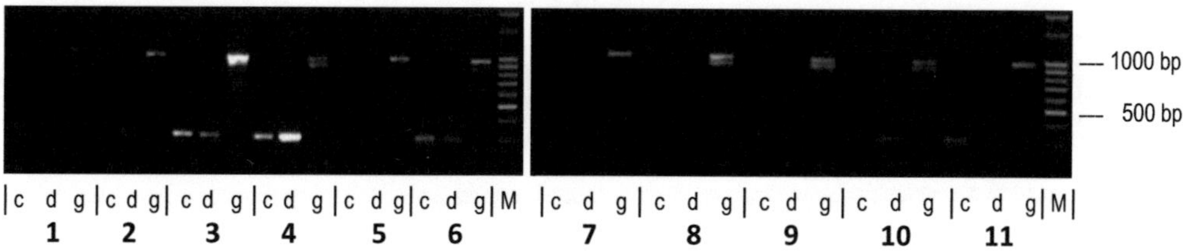

Figure 8. Expression pattern of gene corresponding to BI543243 in sugar beet leaves (c—template cDNA deriving from control plants; d—template cDNA deriving from plants exposed to drought). Amplification on genomic DNA served as additional control (g). M—100 bp DNA ladder size marker.

3.3. Analyses of changes in expression of genes involved in reactions to water stress (plants from greenhouse experiment)

Changes in the expression of 13 candidate genes in 11 different sugar beet genotypes were followed in leaves of plants grown in the greenhouse. Expression pattern corresponding to BI543243 differed in plants exposed to drought in comparison with corresponding controls in genotypes 1, 10, and 11 (**Figure 8**). Therefore, it may serve to develop molecular marker useful to differentiate genotypes with respect to drought.

4. Conclusion

Tolerance to drought is very complex. Experiments in three different environments (tissue culture, greenhouse, and field) with 11 genotypes, where many different parameters were followed, revealed that it is not easy to find single criteria for classification with respect to drought tolerance. However, the results suggest that free proline accumulation may be used as a reliable parameter. The classification based on changes in concentration of free proline in plants exposed to drought in greenhouse and tissue culture corresponded to classification made on the bases on field observations. Therefore, similar fast tests, conducted with young plants and possibly aided by the use of molecular markers, can be useful for estimation of breeding material with respect to tolerance to water deficiency, which will significantly enhance sugar beet breeding for expected future changes in climate.

Acknowledgements

We thank European Union's Horizon 2020 research and innovation program under Grant Agreement No. 691998 and Ministry of Education, Science and Technological Development of the Republic of Serbia for financial support.

Author details

Marina Putnik-Delić[1]*, Ivana Maksimović[1], Nevena Nagl[2] and Branislava Lalić[1]

*Address all correspondence to: putnikdelic@polj.uns.ac.rs

1 Faculty of Agriculture, University of Novi Sad, Novi Sad, Serbia

2 Institute of Field and Vegetable Crops, Novi Sad, Serbia

References

[1] Spasić P. Planiranje prinosa i kvaliteta šećerne repe pri određenim ekološkim uslovima proizvodnje. In: Zbornik radova 16; Poljoprivredni fakultet, Institut za ratarstvo i povrtarstvo; Novi Sad; 1989

[2] Maksimovic L, Dragovic S. Potrebe za vodom i efekat navodnjavanja ratarskih biljaka. In: Zbornik radova X Kongresa JDPZ; Beograd, CD; 2001

[3] Lalic B, Eitzinger J, Mihailovic DT, Thaler S, Jancic M. Climate change impacts on winter wheat yield change—Which climatic parameters are crucial in Pannonian lowland? The Journal of Agricultural Science. 2012;**151**(06):757-774

[4] Kottek M, Grieser J, Beck C, Rudolf B, Rubel F. World map of the Köppen–Geiger climate classification updated. Meteorologische Zeitschrift. 2006;**15**:259-263

[5] Mihailović DT, Lalić B, Drešković N, Mimić G, Djurdjević V, Jančić M. Climate change effects on crop yields in Serbia and related shifts of Köppen climate zones under the SRES-A1B and SRES-A2. International Journal of Climatology. 2015;**35**(11):3320-3334. DOI: 10.1002/joc

[6] Djurdjević V, Rajković B. Development of the EBU-POM coupled regional climate model and results from climate change experiments. In: Mihailović DT, Lalić B, editors. Advances in Environmental Modelling and Measurements. New York: Nova Science Publisher Inc.; 2012. pp. 23-32

[7] Kastori R, Petrović N. Rastenje i razviće šećerne repe. U: Spasić, P, Tošić M, Dokić P, Kastori R, Sekulić R: Šećerna repa, Jugošećer DD, Beograd; 1992. p. 173-189

[8] Fahim MG, Mirzamasoumzadeh B, Ahadzadeh B. Effect of polyethylene glycol on the amount of chlorophyll a, chlorophyll b and total leaf of sugar. Journal of Biodiversity and Environmental Sciences. 2014;**4**(1):233-237 ISSN: 2220-6663 (Print) 2222-3045 (Online)

[9] Силаева AM. Структура хлоропластов и факторы среды. Киев: Наукова Думка; 1978

[10] Dodd IC. Soil moisture heterogeneity during deficit irrigation alters root-to-shoot signaling of abscisic acid. Functional Plant Biology. 2007;**34**:439-448

[11] Qin F, Shinozaki K, Yamaguchi-Shinozaki K. Achievements and challenges in understanding plant abiotic stress responses and tolerance. Plant and Cell Physiology. 2011;**52**:1569-1582

[12] Petrović M, Stikić R. Vodni režim šećerne repe. U: Spasić, P, Tošić M, Dokić P, Kastori R, Sekulić R: Šećerna repa, Jugošećer DD, Beograd; 1992. p. 225-240

[13] Maksimović I, Ćurčić Ž, Nagl N, Kovačev L. Changes in petioles and leaf blades in response to progressive drought in young sugar beet plants. In: XV FESPB Congress, Federation of European Societies of Plant Biology; Lyon, France; 2006. p. 184

[14] Noghabi AM, Williams BF. Drought stress and weed competition in sugar beet. British Sugar Beet Review. 2000;**1**:47-49

[15] Blum A. Plant Breeding for Water-Limited Environments. © Springer Science+Business Media, LLC; New York; 2011. DOI 10.1007/978-1-4419-7491-4_2

[16] Ober ES, Luterbacher MC. Genotypic variation for drought tolerance in Beta Vulgaris. Annals of Botany. 2002;**89**:917-924

[17] Salvucci ME, Crafts-Bradner SJ. Inhibition of photosynthesis by heat stress: The activation state of Rubisco as a limiting factor in photosynthesis. Physiologia Plantarum. 2004;**120**:179-186

[18] Dickison WC. Integrative Plant Anatomy. San Diego: Academic Press; 2000

[19] Thomas T, Clarke N. Are sugar beet problems being watered down? British Sugar Beet Review. 1995;**3**:8-11

[20] Fahn A, Cutler DF. In: Braun HJ, Carlquist S, Ozenda P, Roth I, editors. Xerophytes (Encyclopedia of Plant Anatomy, Vol. XIII, No. 3). Berlin, Stuttgart: Gebruder Borntraeger; 1992

[21] Luković J, Maksimović I, Zorić L, Nagl N, Perčić M, Polić D, Putnik-Delić M. Histological characteristics of sugar beet leaves potentially linked to drought tolerance. Industrial Crops and Products. 2009;**30**:281-286

[22] Du J, Chen X, Li W, Gao Q. Osmoregulation mechanism of drought stress and genetic engineering strategies for improving drought resistance in plants. Forestry Studies in China. 2004;**6**(2):56-62

[23] Huang X, Wei X, Sang T, Zhao Q, Feng Q, Zhao Y, Li C, Zhu C, Lu T, Zhang Z, Li M, Fan D, Guo Y, Wang A, Wang L, Deng L, Li W, Lu Y, Weng Q, Liu K, Huang T, Zhou T, Jing Y, Li W, Lin Z. Genome-wide association studies of 14 agronomic traits in rice landraces. Nature Genetics. 2010;**42**:961-967

[24] Nayyar H, Walia DP. Water stress induced proline accumulation in contrasting wheat genotypes as affected by calcium and abscisic acid. Biologia Plantarum. 2003;**46**(2):275-279

[25] DeRonde JA, Spreeth MH, Cress WA. Effect of antisense pxrroline-5carboxylate reductase transgenic soybean plants subjected to osmotic and drought stress. Plant Growth Regulation. 2000;**32**:13-26

[26] Conde A, Chaves MM, Geros H. Membrane transport, sensing and signaling in plant adaptation to environmental stress. Plant and Cell Physiology. 2011;**52**(9):1583-1602

[27] Valliyodan B, Nguyen H. Understanding regulatory networks and engineering for enhanced drought tolerance in plants. Current Opinion in Plant Biology. 2006;**9**:189-195

[28] Putnik-Delić M, Maksimović I, Venezia A, Nagl N. Free proline accumulation in young sugar beet plants and in tissue culture explants under water deficiency as tools for assessment of drought tolerance. Romanian Agricultural Research. 2013;**30**:141-148

[29] Monreal JA, Jimenez ET, Remesal E, Morillo-Velarde S, Garcia- Maurino S, Echevarria C. Proline content of sugar beet storage roots: Response to water deficit and nitrogen fertilization at field conditions. Environmental and Experimental Botany. 2007;**60**(2):257-267

[30] Coca M, Garcıa MT, Gonzalez G, Pena M, Garcıa JA. Study of coloured components formed in sugar beet processing. Food Chemistry. 2004;**86**:421-433

[31] Hoai NTT, Shim IS, Kobayashi K, Kenji U. Accumulation of some nitrogen compounds in response to salt stress and their relationships with salt tolerance in rice (*Oryza sativa* L.) seedlings. Plant Growth Regulation. 2003;**41**:159-164

[32] Szabados L, Savouré A. Proline: A multifunctional amino acid. Trends in Plant Science. 2009;**15**(2):89-97

[33] Feuillet C, Langridge P, Waugh R. Cereal breeding takes a walk on the wild side. Trends in Genetics. 2008;**24**:24-32

[34] Honma Y, Taguchi K, Hiyama H, Yui-Kurino R, Mikami T, Kubo T. Molecular mapping of restorer-of-fertility 2 gene identified from a sugar beet (*Beta vulgaris* L. ssp. vulgaris) homozygous for the non-restoring restorer-of-fertility 1 allele. Theoretical and Applied Genetics. 2014;**127**(12):2567-2574. DOI: 10.1007/s00122-014-2398-4

[35] Whitmore AP, Whalley WR. Physical effects of soil drying on roots and crop growth. Journal of Experimental Botany. 2009;**60**:2845-2857

[36] Neumann PM. Coping mechanisms for crop plants in drought-prone environments. Annals of Botany. 2008;**101**:901-907

[37] Würschum T, Reif JC, Kraft T, Janssen G, Zhao Y. Genomic selection in sugar beet breeding populations. BMC Genetics. 2013;**14**:85. DOI: 10.1186/1471-2156-14-85

[38] Collins NC, Tardieu F, Tuberosa R. Quantitative trait loci and crop performance under abiotic stress: Where do we stand? Plant Physiology. 2008;**147**:469-486

[39] Ries D, Holtgräwe D, Viehöver P, Weisshaar B. Rapid gene identification in sugar beet using deep sequencing of DNA from phenotypic pools selected from breeding panels. BMC Genomics. 2016;**17**:236. DOI: 10.1186/s12864-016-2566-9

[40] Chaves MM, Flexas J, Pinheiro C. Photosynthesis under drought and salt stress: Regulation mechanisms from whole plant to cell. Annals of Botany. 2009;**103**:551-560

[41] Nakashiama K, Ito Y, Yamaguchi-Shinozaki K. Transcriptional regulatory networks in response to abiotic stresses in Arabidopsis and grasses. Plant Physiology. 2009;**149**:88-95

[42] Putnik-Delić M. Physiological and molecular aspects of sugar beet tolerance to drought [PhD thesis]. Novi Sad: University of Novi Sad, Faculty of Agriculture; 2013. p. 125

[43] Bates LS. Rapid determination of free proline for water-stress studies. Plant and Soil. 1973;**39**:205-207

[44] Holm G. Chlorophyll mutations in barley. Acta Agriculturae Scandinavica. 1954;**4**:457-471

[45] Wettstein D von. Chlorophyll-letale und der submikroskopische Formwechsel der Plastiden. Experimental Cell Research 1975;**12**:427-506

[46] Murashige T, Skoog F. A revised medium for growth and bioassays with tobacco tissue cultures. Physiologia Plantarum. 1962;**15**:473-497

[47] De los Reyes BG, McGrath JM, Myers S, Derrico C. Differential Gene Expression in Sugar Beet Seedlings (*Beta vulgaris*) Germinated Under Stress Conditions. 2000. http://www.ncbi.nlm.nih.gov/nucest/

[48] De los Reyes BG, McGrath JM, Myers S. Differential Gene Expression in Sugar Beet Seedlings (*Beta vulgaris*) Germinated Under Stress Conditions. 2001. http://www.ncbi.nlm.nih.gov/nucest/

[49] De los Reyes BG, McGrath JM, Myers S, Trebbi D. Expressed Sequence Tags of *Beta vulgaris*. 2001. http://www.ncbi.nlm.nih.gov/nucest/

[50] Close TJ, Kortt AA, Chandler PM. A cDNA-based comparison of dehydration-induced proteins (dehydrins) in barley and corn. Journal of Plant Molecular Biology. 1989;**13**(1):95-108

[51] Hadfield J. Metode MCMC methods for multi-response generalized linear mixed models: MCMCglmm R paket. Journal of Statistical Software. 2010;**33**(2):1-22

[52] Development Core R, Team R. A Language and Environment for Statistical Computing. Vienna, Austria: R Foundation for Statistical Computing; 2012. http://www.R-project.org

[53] Bates D, Maechler M, Bolker B. lme4: Linear Mixed-Effects Models Using S4 Classes. R Package Version 0.999375-42. 2011. http://CRAN.Rproject.org/package=lme4

[54] Wickham H. ggplot2: Elegant Graphics for Data Analysis. New York: Springer; 2009

[55] Putnik-Delic M, Maksimovic I, Djoric E, Nagl N. Analyses of statistical transformations of row data describing free proline concentration in sugar beet exposed to drought. Matica Srpska, Proceedings for Natural Sciences. 2010;**119**:7-16

[56] Liu W, He Y, Xiang J, Fu C, Yu L, Zhang J, Li M. The physiological response of suspension cell of *Capparis spinosa* L. to drought stress. Journal of Medicinal Plant Research. 2011;**5**(24):5899-5906

Chapter 5

Transcriptome, Genetic Transformation and Micropropagation: Some Biotechnology Strategies to Diminish Water Stress Caused by Climate Change in Sugarcane

Evelyn Arlette Carrillo Bermejo,
Miguel Angel Herrera Alamillo,
Samuel David Gamboa Tuz,
Miguel Angel Keb Llanes,
Enrique Castaño de la Serna, Manuel L. Robert and
Luis Carlos Rodríguez Zapata

Additional information is available at the end of the chapter

http://dx.doi.org/10.5772/intechopen.72438

Abstract

Global climate change caused by natural processes results in major environmental issues that affect the world. Climate variability results in changes that cause water stress in plants. Sugarcane is a tropical grass C4, perennial and a multi-purpose industrial cash crop which serves as the main source of raw material for the production of sugar and biofuel. Farmers face the challenge to provide biotech alternatives with potential benefits and minimize potential adverse impacts on sugarcane's production. In order to find biotechnology strategies to diminish the impact of climate change, our laboratory teamworks with micropropagation, transcriptome and genetic transformation of sugarcane using the var. MEX69290. In the transcriptome of sugarcane, a total of 536 and 750 genes were differentially regulated under normal and water stress treatment respectively, of which key genes were selected to be inserted into sugarcane for tolerance to abiotic stress. Regarding results of micropropagation, it was concluded that the continuous immersion propagation system was the best culture strategy. This may be as result of the elimination of gelling agent, which additionally helps reduce production costs.

Keywords: biotechnology, micropropagation systems, transcriptome, genetic transformation, sugarcane, abiotic stress

1. Introduction

Climate change alters environmental conditions and therefore has direct and biophysical effects on agricultural production. The biophysical and direct effects of climate change induce alterations on the prices and production of agriculture. Such changes are reflected on the economic system as farmers and other market participants make adjustments autonomously. They are both compelled to modify their crop combinations, use of supplies, level of production, and food demand, consumption and trade. Climate change causes a changes in rainfall regimes which have direct effects on crop yields as well as indirect effects through changes in the availability of water irrigation [1].

Sugarcane (*Saccharum officinarum* L.) is a monocotyledonous perennial plant belonging to the gramineous family *Saccharum officinarum* L. [2]. Sugarcane is a commercial crop in tropical and subtropical regions. According to FAOSTAT [3], sugarcane is cultivated in 26.1 million hectares producing 1.83 trillion canes. Sugarcane is a multi-purpose industrial cash crop and the main source of raw material for sugar production. It is responsible for almost 70% of world-produced centrifugal sugar [4]. Some mitigation and adaptation strategies for climate change in sugarcane production are the use of biotechnological techniques such as transcriptome, genetic transformation and *in vitro* micropropagation. In this chapter, we will talk about water stress in sugarcane caused by the climatic change and the biotechnological alternatives such as transcriptome, genetic transformation and micropropagation which are currently being carried out in our laboratory to counteract this problem.

2. Climate change, water stress and its effect in sugarcane

A large scale of plant production grown under different agricultural production systems is lost under the effects of abiotic stresses, which may result in a 70% reduction of the potential yields of crop plants [5]. During growth and developmental periods, crops suffer seasonal floods and droughts, extreme temperatures or salinity all year round. Globally, about 22% of global agricultural land is saline, and the increased damage caused by drought has been reported to limit plant growth and development followed by a loss of productivity, especially in crop species [6, 7]. Thus, drought stresses are one of the most serious kind of abiotic stresses that implies a threat on crop productivity worldwide.

Sugarcane, an important source of sugar and ethanol, is a relatively high water-demanding crop and its growth is highly sensitive to water deficit [8]. It is estimated that sugarcane produces 8–12 ton cane per ML of water irrigation [9], and water deficit can lead to productivity losses of up to 60% [10–13]. For this reason, production areas are concentrated in regions with favorable rain regime to sugarcane growth and development [14], while in other areas crop production requires supplemental or full irrigation [15].

According to various studies, water stress triggers many physiological, biochemical, and molecular responses that influence various cellular processes in plants and this impacts on its productivity [16, 17].

Severe water stress such as drought affects the entire plant. Morphological and physiological responses in sugarcane plants vary according to its genotype, duration (rapid or gradual) and intensity (severe or mild) of stress and also the type of affected tissue [18–21]. Water stress also affects both cane and sugar yield substantially. The most common water stress responses in sugarcane are leaf rolling, stomatal closure, inhibition of stalk and leaf growth, leaf senescence and reduced leaf area [12, 22]. Moreover, under water stress, both cell division and cell elongation are interrupted [23] and stem and leaf elongation are the most severely affected growth processes [24, 25]. Root development is also influenced by water deficit [19, 26] but its overall biomass is relatively less than the above-ground biomass. Sugarcane is a tropical crop with C4 photosynthetic metabolism. A moderate water stress causes a stomatal limitation, which triggers a decrease in stomatal conductance (gs), transpiration rate (E), internal CO_2 concentration (Ci), and photosynthetic rate [26–30]. Under water stress, a decline in photosynthetic rate is mainly caused by a decrease in phosphoenolpyruvate carboxylase (PEPcase) and ribulose-1,5-biphosphate carboxylase (Rubisco) activity [26, 27, 31]. It is worth to note that photosynthesis rate is also impacted by sugar accumulation in leaves [32]. Under non-stressed condition low leaf sugar content is conducive to photosynthesis, while high sugar content moderates carbon fixation [33]. Interestingly, increased levels of some sugars, such as trehalose, can help plants to cope with water deficit, reducing the damage on cell membrane [34]. The capacity to accumulate trehalose was demonstrated in sugarcane roots under drought conditions. Sales et al. [35] reported an increase in starch hydrolysis, leading to higher levels of soluble sugars that helped sustain carbon supply even in a reduced CO_2 fixation condition, facilitating growth recovery after stress.

3. Sugarcane and biotechnology

Sugarcane crop productivity has progressively increased to remarkable levels worldwide in the last century [36]. This increase in productivity has been ascribed to the development and widespread use of improved cultivars with increased resistance to diseases and pests, better management of water, nutrients and other resources, and the availability of relatively cheap chemical fertilizers and pesticides. Sustaining this pace of improvement in crop productivity by innovative and intensive agriculture, whilst ensuring minimal environmental impact, will be one of the major challenges to maintain a profitable sugar industry in the future.

Biotechnology offers excellent opportunities for sugarcane crop improvement. Commercial sugarcane, mainly the interspecific hybrids of *S. officinarum* and *S. spontaneum* [37], would greatly benefit from biotechnological improvements due to its complex polyploid-aneuploid genome, narrow genetic base, poor fertility, susceptibility to various diseases and pests, and the long duration (12–15 years) required to breed elite cultivars. More importantly, there is an ongoing need to provide durable disease and pest resistance commercial clones in combination with superior agronomic performance. This led to considerable research in different areas of biotechnology pertinent to sugarcane breeding and disease control. Despite the availability of molecular tools and strategies and advancements in our understanding of stress responses, engineering crops for drought tolerance remains a major challenge. This is not only due to the complexity of the plant responses to water deficit but also due to the difficulty of identifying and exploiting of large effect genes and alleles and the associated selection traits for developing drought tolerant varieties suitable for commercial crop production conditions [38].

4. Micropropagation an alternative to develop plants tolerant to water stress "hyperhydricity"

Various micropropagation systems such as liquid cultures and automation have proven the potential to resolve manual handling of *in vitro* cultures at various stages and decrease production cost. However, hyperhydricity is a major problem during *in vitro* culture of many crops in liquid culture systems. Hyperhydricity (also known as "vitrification") is a physiological disorder occurring in plant material of tissue culture, which causes a reduction of propagation and death of tissues when transferred to *ex vitro* conditions [39–41]. The environment inside culture vessels normally used for plant micropropagation is characterized by high humidity, limited gaseous exchange between the internal atmosphere of the culture vessel and its surrounding environment, and the accumulation of ethylene; conditions that may induce physiological disorders [42]. The development of hyperhydric deformities represents a disadvantage for plant micropropagation and a barrier for the exploitation of bioreactor technologies to scale-up its production [41]. The concept of stress in relation to hyperhydricity is not completely established. Therefore, it remains difficult to assume when hyperhydric tissues are stressed. Previous studies argued that abnormal morphology observed in hyperhydricity could be attributed to changes occurring at cellular level due to the modifications of membrane composition or DNA content [42]. However, Rojas-Martínez and coworkers [41] considered this disorder as the result of the stressful conditions brought out by waterlogging of the apoplast. This causes hypoxia and thereby leads to severe oxidative stress. They concluded that hyperhydric features like vitreous appearance and wrinkled leaves are secondary events resulting from waterlogging of the apoplast.

The temporary immersion system (TIS) consists on the use of bioreactors with automated devices that control features such as gas exchange, liquid medium culture and lighting, required for the growth, development and survival of plants. TIS mainly consist of three phases: multiplication, elongation and rooting phase. Plantlets propagated in TIS have better performance than those propagated by conventional methods of micropropagation. TIS provides a rapid and efficient plant propagation system for many agricultural and forestry species, it utilizes liquid media avoiding intensive manual handling [43].

With the objective of evaluating the stress caused by hyperhydricity in the *in vitro* culture of sugarcane var. MEX69290, three types of culture were analyzed: Semisolid (Magenta) was used as control; Continuous immersion (250 ml Flask); and Temporary Immersion (BioMINT II Bioreactor). Multiplication, maturation, and *ex vitro* adaptation phases of sugarcane under these three types of culture were evaluated.

The obtained results in the adaptation of *in vitro* plants of *S. officinarum* at three different types of culture in the multiplication phase were surprising, as it is observed in **Figure 1**, where a notorious formation of shoots occurs in continuous immersion medium. Plants of var. MEX69290 obtained a much higher average shoot formation at the temporary immersion bioreactors than those observed in semi-solid medium. It was observed that invariable of the inoculum density applied (5, 10, 15 plants per bottle) was higher in continuous immersion. Similarly, growth index factor was higher in this culture system than that obtained in semi-solid medium or temporary immersion bioreactors (**Figure 1**). We can observe comparing our results with other works that the treatment response depends on the type of explant and variety of sugarcane. Several studies have reported that the rate of shoot formation is higher in temporary immersion bioreactors than in semi-solid cultures. It is important to mention that none of the previous works reported any problem with the hyperhydricity in the obtained *in vitro* plants. Only, Snyman [44] reports this condition on the induction and germination of somatic sugarcane embryos. Tesfa and coworkers [45], didn't report problems of hyperhydricity or a decrease in field survival rate out of *in vitro* plants after using a liquid culture medium with agitation

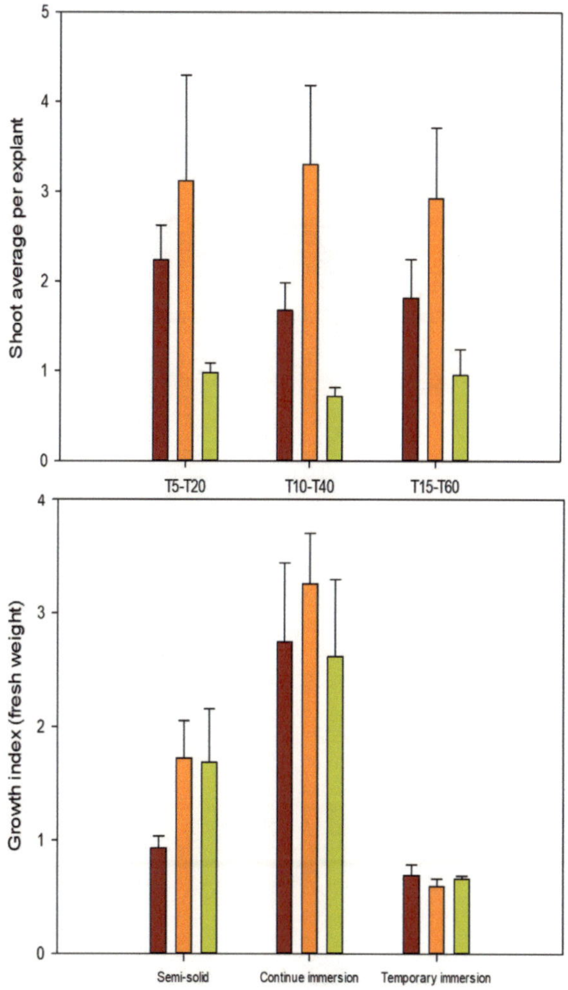

Figure 1. Average of shoots at different densities of inoculum. T5-T20: 5 inoculum plants were used in semi-solid and continuous immersion medium, 20 plants in temporary immersion; T10-T40: 10 inoculum plants were used in semi-solid and continuous immersion medium, and 40 plants in temporary immersion; T15-T60: 15 inoculum plants were used in semi-solid and continuous immersion medium, and 60 plants in temporary immersion; semisolid (red rectangle), continue immersion (orange rectangle) and temporary immersion (green rectangle). At the bottom of the figure, the calculated growth index factor is reported using the obtained fresh weight under the same inoculum density conditions; T5-T20 (red rectangle), T10-T40 (orange rectangle) and T15-T60 (green rectangle). Five replicates were carried out for each treatment.

(80 rpm) in which they obtained an average shoot emission of 6.95 and 6.30 in the two cultivars used. The shoot emissions and growing index of the sugarcane variety MEX69290 was not affected when cultivated in a stationary liquid medium for 28 days (**Figure 1**).

The variety MEX69290 clones' response at the maturation phase showed the same behavior as that observed at the multiplication phase, with the average shoot emission and the growth index being higher in the liquid culture than the one obtained in half semi-solid or in the temporary immersion bioreactor culture (**Figure 2**).

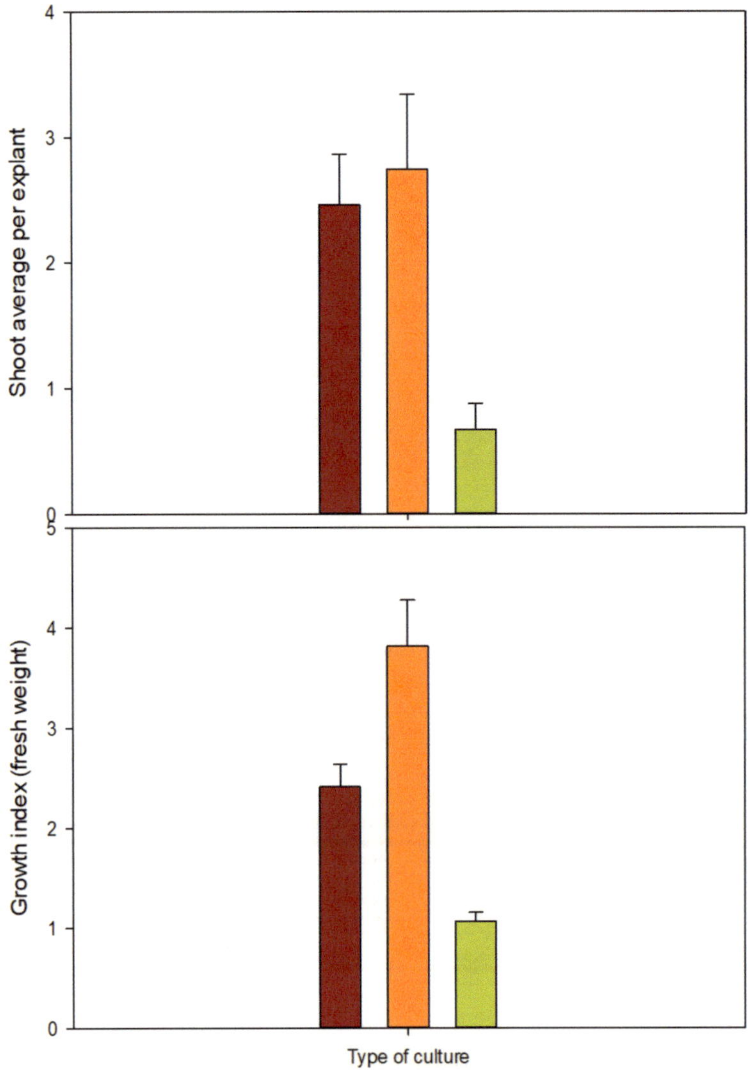

Figure 2. Mean of shoots using 10 in vitro plants in semi-solid and continuous immersion cultures and 60 plants in temporary immersion bioreactors. At the bottom of the figure the calculated growth index factor is reported using the obtained fresh weight under the same inoculum density conditions. Five replicates were carried out for each treatment. Semisolid (red rectangle), continue immersion (orange rectangle) and temporary immersion (green rectangle).

After 28 days in maturation phase, 120 plants from semi-solid culture, 120 plants under continuous immersion, and 75 from BIOMINT were adapted. In **Figure 3**, we can observe the quality of the plants from the same clone at the three different cultivation systems.

Plants underwent a 28 days preadaptation period, and afterward were planted and placed in greenhouse conditions. Once plants where transferred into the greenhouse, their survival rate was evaluated, being 100% in all cases (**Figure 4**). Plants from the temporary immersion bioreactors were taller and with longer leaves, but those from semi-solid medium and continuous immersion continued to emit shoots during the following 4 months evaluation at the greenhouse. The results obtained in this phase are very similar to those reported by Arencibia et al. [46], Bernal et al. [47], and Silva et al. [48], who reported survival rates higher than 96% in the different cultivars using a temporary immersion bioreactor, and our result is much higher than the studies reported by Snyman et al. [44], with only 34% of survival rate from sugarcane grown in the RITA system.

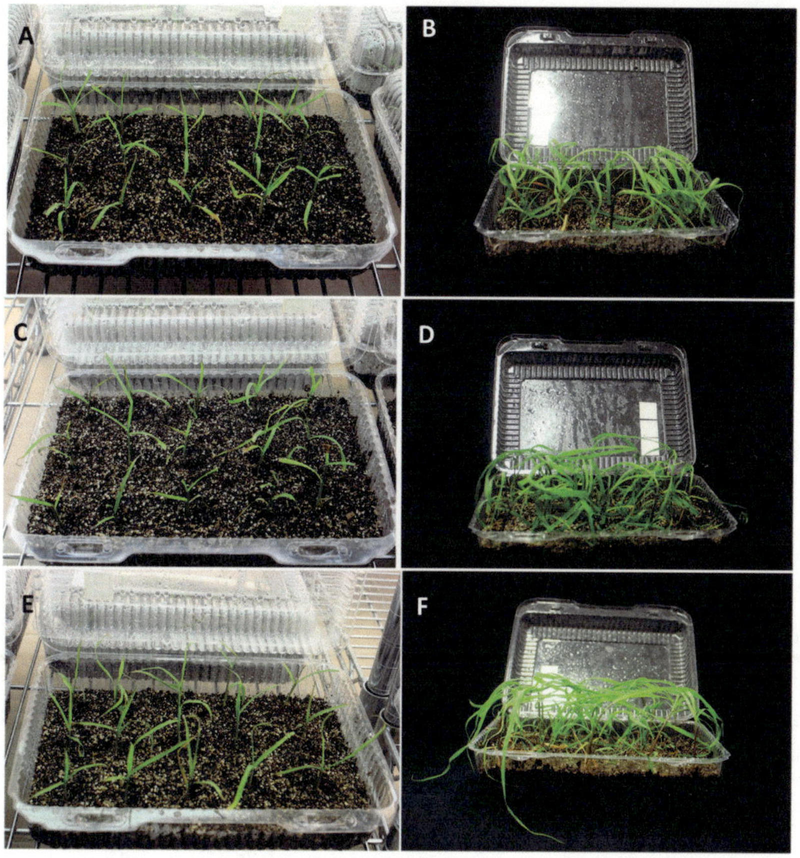

Figure 3. Phase adaptation of *in vitro* plants of *S. officinarum* var. MEX69290, seeded in a germination mixture BM2, previously autoclaved. 15 plants per container were adapted in growth culture room at 25°C with 16/8 hours photoperiod light/dark. (A) and (B) day zero and twenty-eight, of plants coming from semi-solid culture; (C) and (D) day zero and twenty-eight, of plants coming from liquid culture; (E) and (F) day zero and twenty-eight, of plants coming from temporary immersion system (BioMINT).

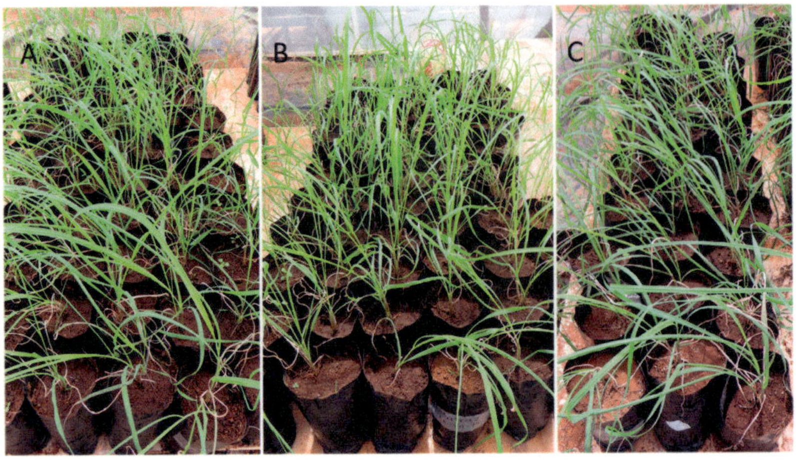

Figure 4. Greenhouse adaptation of *in vitro* plants of *S. officinarum* var. MEX69290, from culture: (A) semi-solid; (B) continuous immersion; (C) temporary immersion. Substrate consisted on a 3: 1 mixture of sunshine: soil. All plantlets survived 100% after 30 days in the greenhouse.

The best results out of the measured parameters were obtained from the continuous immersion propagation system. It was concluded the reason for this may reside in the elimination of gelling agent, which additionally lowers production costs in the process of delivering this sugarcane's variety to the field. Plants obtained under this system achieved normal development, they developed shoots and roots cyclically and no vitrification was detected in any of the evaluated micropropagation phases. This suggests that the clone obtained from the MEX69290 variety is tolerant to liquid culture conditions. Apparently this system does not generate an abiotic stress, stationing it as a prospective medium to perform genetic transformation processes and to study its gene expression pattern that could further make enhanced tolerant clones.

5. Transcriptomic analysis of an elite Mexican sugarcane cultivar ('Mex 69-290') in response to osmotic stress. Identification of genes with biotechnological potential

Modern sugarcane cultivars have been obtained by inter-specific hybridizations between the high-sucrose-yielding of *S. officinarum* (2n = 8x = 80) and the stress-tolerant *S. spontaneum* (2n = 40–128). As a consequence, sugarcane cultivars present large (10 Gb) and poly-aneuploid genomes with numerous gene alleles and repetitive sequences. Such genome complexity has made it difficult to obtain a complete sequenced reference genome that could aid in the identification of novel genes with biotechnological potential for the improvement of this important C4 crop. Alternatively, de novo transcriptome assembly of reads produced by high-throughput sequencing technologies (also referred to as Next Generation Sequencing (NGS)) offers a mean to unravel global gene expression changes in response to various conditions in sugarcane. For example, some recent works have employed High-throughput sequencing to identify sugarcane genes involved in leaf abscission [49], biomass content and composition [50], and abiotic stress [51]. Li and cols. [49] performed a transcriptome analysis to identify genes associated with leaf abscission in sugarcane. They employed the Illumina HiSeq 2000 platform (2x90pb) to analyze six cDNA libraries from parents and their F1 offspring, which present different leaf abscission behaviors. After a total assembly, they found 275,018 transcripts corresponding to 164,803 genes. Then, to identify genes related to leaf abscission in sugarcane [49], analyzed a core set of 1, 202 transcripts which were up-regulated in leaf abscission sugarcane plants (LASP) in comparison to leaf packaging sugarcane plants (LPSP). They found that some of these genes were associated with plant-pathogen interaction, response to stress, and ABA-associated pathways. On the other hand [50], performed an extensive transcriptome analysis to identify genes associated with biomass content. They employed the Illumina HiSeq 4000 platform to analyze cDNA libraries from 20 internodal samples of 10 different sugarcane genotypes, which were divided in low and high fiber containing groups. They found 5601 and 4659 unique expressed transcripts in High and Low fiber containing genotypes; and 83,421 shared expressed transcripts between both groups. Furthermore, they found 555 differentially expressed transcripts between low and high fiber containing genotypes. Of these, 151 and 23 transcripts corresponded to sugar and fiber accumulation, respectively. Some of these genes were involved in Carbohydrate metabolism, Photosynthesis, Cell-wall metabolism and Lignin Pathway; DIR proteins were also represented [50].

Regarding abiotic stress, Belesini and cols. [51] analyzed the transcriptomic profile of the drought-tolerant 'SP81-3250' and the drought-sensitive 'RB855453' sugarcane cultivars under drought stress conditions for 30, 60, and 90 days. They analyzed a total of 54 cDNA libraries by Illumina HiScanSQ System and HiSeq 2500 platforms. Among the genes that were induced in the drought-tolerant cultivar, they found an ascorbate peroxidase, a MYB TF, an E3 SUMO-protein ligase SIZ2, a coenzyme A ligase (a key enzyme for the biosynthesis of flavonoids), and an aquaporin, among others. These types of genes are well known to play a role in abiotic stress tolerance. In the drought-sensitive cultivar they found several kinases that were induced upon stress like Receptor like protein kinases (RLK), which might play a role in stress stimulus perception; bHLH transcription factors; ACC oxidase from the ethylene biosynthetic pathway; and many undescribed genes. More recently (2017), in our laboratory Pereira-Santana and cols. [52] analyzed the transcriptomic profile of the 2nd most important sugarcane cultivar in Mexico, 'Mex 69-290', in response to osmotic stress. In such study, authors employed the High-throughput sequencing system HiSeq-Illumina (2x100bp) to analyze 16 cDNA libraries representing leaves and roots of *in vitro*-grown plantlets exposed to PEG-8000 during 0, 24, 48, and 72 hours. After assembly of a total of 140, 339 unigenes, Pereira-Santana and cols. Found core sets of 536 and 750 up-regulated genes in response to osmotic stress in roots and leaves, respectively; and core sets of 1093 and 531 down-regulated genes in roots and leaves, respectively. After gene annotation, the authors found that sugarcane 'MEX69290' responds to osmotic stress by increasing the expression of genes involved in transcription regulation, oxide-reduction, carbohydrate catabolism, and flavonoid and other secondary metabolites biosynthesis. Genes responsive to ABA, water deprivation, and heat stress were also up-regulated. On the other hand, this sugarcane cultivar responds to osmotic stress by decreasing the expression of genes involved in sucrose and starch metabolic processes, cell wall biogenesis, cellulose biosynthesis, anion transport, and light response. A handful of the genes found by Pereria-Santana and cols. Are presented along with their expression profiles in the heat map of **Figure 5A**. Because of the well-defined expression pattern of some of these genes, they could prove to be useful as expression markers in the response of 'MEX69290' to osmotic stress. For example, ABA 8-hydroxylase 3, Isoflavone 2-hydroxylase, LEA 14A, and NAC TF 25 showed clear patterns of up-regulation. In fact, in our laboratory further expression and functional analyses are currently being carried out regarding this NAC TF25 gene. Conversely, Bidirectional sugar transporter SWEET11, Cellulose synthase E6, and Sugar transporter ERD6 16 showed clear patterns of down-regulation. These down-regulated genes are also interesting, not just because of their responsiveness to osmotic stress but also due to their involvement in sucrose metabolism. The engineering of these genes might increase biomass production in sugarcane and tolerance to osmotic stress simultaneously. Furthermore, many TFs known to play important roles in the stress responses of plants, i.e. HSF, ZN, bZIP, WRKY, NAC, and MYB, were found in abundance in the total assembly of the 'MEX69290' transcriptome (**Figure 5B**). Even when some of these TF families seemed underrepresented (like NAC and MYC), they still provide a useful benchmark to conduct phylogenetic, expression, and functional analysis.

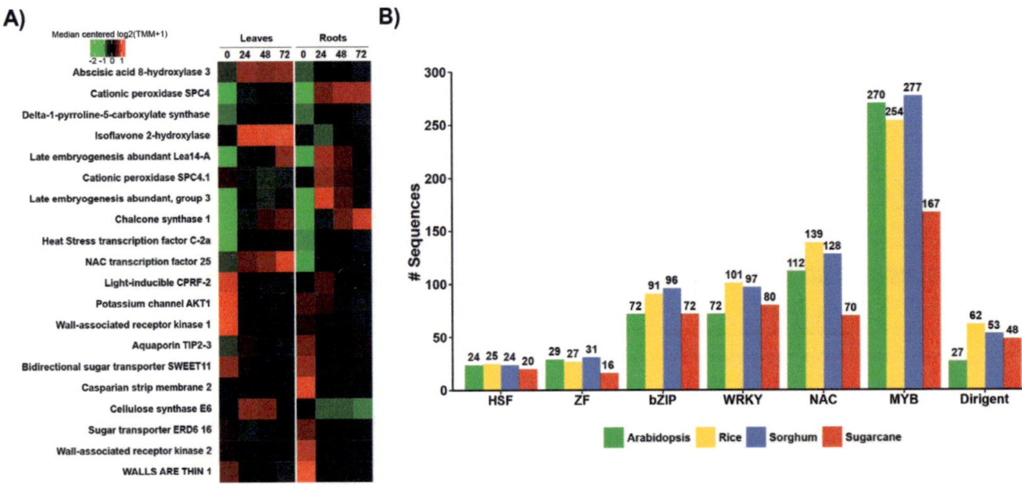

Figure 5. Selected DEGs in response to osmotic stress and abundance of major TF families and Dirigent protein family in sugarcane 'MEX69290' transcriptome. (A) Expression profile of 20 selected DEGs in leaves and roots of sugarcane 'MEX69290' plantlets submitted to PEG-8000 treatment during 0, 24, 48, and 72 hours. Data was obtained from the work of Pereira-Santana and cols [52]. The heat map was generated with the ComplexHeatmappackage v1.14.0 [52] in R v3.4.1 [53]. (B) Abundance of major stress-related TF families and Dirigent protein family in arabidopsis, rice, sorghum, and sugarcane. The results were obtained by means of HMM searches using the profiles of the HSF (PF00447), ZF (PF00096), bZIP (PF00170), WRKY (PF03106), NAC (PF02365), MYB (PF00249), and Dirigent (PF03018) proteins obtained from the Pfam database (http://pfam.xfam.org) [54]. For this analysis the complete predicted proteomes (primary transcripts only) of arabidopsis, rice, and sorghum were obtained from Phytozome v. 12 [55]. Sugarcane predicted protein dataset was obtained from the transcriptome assembly of Pereira-Santana and cols [52] HMM searches were performed using HMMER3 v3.1b2 (http://hmmer.org/) and set to a cut-off e-value of 1e-05 and a score above the inclusion threshold of each HMM profile.

In addition to the insights about the global gene expression dynamics of 'Mex 69-290' in response to osmotic stress and the identification of novel TFs, the work of Pereira-Santana and cols. Provides a useful benchmark for the study of other specific gene families of biotechnological significance for sugarcane engineering, for example the DIR protein family. Plant DIR proteins are believed to be involved in lignin biosynthesis, defense [56, 57], and abiotic stress responses such as dehydration [58], and salinity and oxidative stress [59]. In a recent study, 5 available sequence databases for sugarcane were surveyed, a total of 120 DIR proteins were identified [60]. Phylogenetic analysis showed that these DIR proteins are divided in 64 groups and 7 major clades: Dir-a, Dir-b/d, Dir-c, Dir-e, Dir-g, Dir-h, and Dir-i [60]. In the sugarcane transcriptome assembly of 'sugarcane Mex 69-290' performed in our laboratory by Pereira-Santana and cols, a total of 48 predicted proteins with DIR-like domains were identified. These DIR proteins were clustered in 7 groups according to their expression patterns (**Figure 6**). DIR42 protein from cluster 1 was significantly up-regulated in all time points of osmotic stress in root tissues. Conversely, DIR40 protein from cluster 7 was significantly down-regulated in all time points of osmotic stress in leaf tissues. In general, DIR genes from cluster 4 seem to possess a relative high expression in roots under control conditions, and those from cluster 7 seem to possess a relative high expression in leaves under control conditions. DIR genes from both clusters are down-regulated in response to osmotic stress. On the other hand, we also recovered a homolog of the ScDir gene (GenBank: JQ622282.1) from the sugarcane variety FN39 (DIR38 in cluster 5). The expression of ScDir from FN39 has been

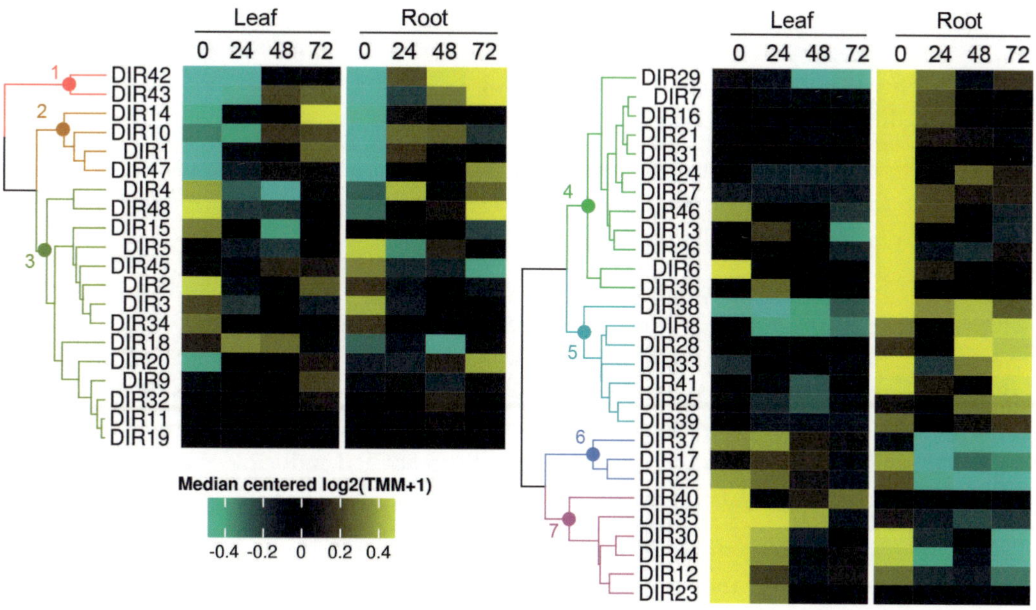

Figure 6. Differential expression in response to osmotic stress of 48 Dirigent proteins found in sugarcane 'MEX69290' transcriptome. The 48 Dirigent sequences from sugarcane were grouped according to their expression profiles in 7 clusters (1–7). Data was obtained from Pereira-Santana and cols [52]. Heat map and sequence clustering were generated with ComplexHeatmap v1.14.0 [53] in R v3.4.1 [54] using the "euclidean" distance method and "complete" clustering method.

reported to be up-regulated in response to H_2O_2, NaCl, and PEG treatment [59]. Furthermore, its heterologous expression in *Escherichia coli* increases the bacterial host's tolerance to NaCl and PEG [59]. The homolog of this gene in 'Mex 69-290' was slightly up-regulated in leaves, but down-regulated in roots (**Figure 6**, cluster 5). All of these mentioned DIR genes from sugarcane 'MEX69290' are interesting because they show differential expression patterns in leaves and roots in response to osmotic stress. However, their functional roles in osmotic stress tolerance and biomass accumulation still need to be experimentally analyzed. In summary, in the absence of a complete sequenced genome for sugarcane, high-throughput sequencing technologies applied to the elucidation of elite cultivars' transcriptome profile are one of the most valuable resources for the identification of genes involved in both stress tolerance and biomass accumulation, which are important agronomic traits to face global climate change.

6. Genetic transformation of cane, a very powerful biotechnological tool to generate tolerant plants to water stress

According to the International Service for the Acquisition of Agri-biotech Applications (ISAAA), the worldwide distribution of genetically modified crops involves a total of 26 developing countries and 7 industrialized countries, headed by USA, Brazil, Argentina, Canada, India, China and South Africa. There is a current approval on the use of two commercial varieties of genetically modified cane in Brazil and Indonesia. On the former, plants containing the Cry1Ab gene, which produces an insecticidal toxin capable of killing the *Diatraea* caterpillar, are being cultivated. In Indonesia plants transformed with the EcBetA gene are resistant to drought.

Scientific research in genetic transformation have focused on resistance to biotic and abiotic factors such as weed control, production of renewable primary products, energy crops and production of pharmaceutically active substances.

Some of the methods in genetic transformation of plants are by Agrobacterium or biolistic which are time consuming, laborious and have low transformation efficiency. Thus we have attempted different options to optimize genetic transformation in sugar cane. An option for efficient transformation is by using different types of vectors, for example Anderson & Birch [61] used Binary super vectors in addition of different types of promoters (constitutive and inducible). Niu et al. [62] is other case who used the SoCINI inducible promoters and the ScMybRI constitutive promoters respectively [62, 63].

On the other hand, different *in vitro* culture protocols have been tried for decades to optimize the efficiency (time and management of the explant) as well as the number of transgenic plants. Yogesh and collaborators transformed cane leaves by Biolistic [64], regenerating seedlings via direct (ED) and indirect (EI) embryogenesis [65]. Arencibia and Carmona [66] reported genetic transformation by *Agrobacterium tumefaciens* and via indirect morphogenesis resulting in regenerated seedlings. Manickavasagam et al. reported regenerated seedlings after *A. tumefaciens* transformation via axillary shoots [67]. These latter two protocols require a time lapse between 3 and 6 months to generate seedlings.

In contrast, a genetic transformation protocol using *A. tumefaciens* has been developed in our laboratory (in the process of obtaining patent) where *in vitro* basal micro-shoots of MEX69290 cultivars underwent the insertion of the CpRap2.4b gene from the AP2/ERF transcription factor family, and out of cDNA of papaya stressed at 40°C. This genetic transformation protocol requires only 20 minutes and has a contamination rate of 0%, as well as a 21-day seedling regeneration rate. Our results showed a 70% survival in the first subculture and 100% in the second subculture with Kanamycin; similar results were reported by Manickavasagam regenerating transgenic seedlings using micro axillary outbreaks out of field plants [67], with a very laborious genetic transformation system and with 50% survival in the first crop. In addition, this work would be the second in sugarcane to report a gene of the AP2/ERF family of transcription factors inserted in sugar cane, the other work is the one reported by Reis et al. where they over expressed AtDREB2A CA (constitutive activity) in sugar cane [68]. In the transformed sugarcane seedlings generated by the genetic transformation protocol that was developed in our laboratory, the presence of the GFP was observed at the fluorescent emission of 395–475 nm, which indicates that the seedlings are transformed (**Figure 7**).

It should be clarified that the functionality of the CpRap2.4b gene belonging to the (AP2/ERF) transcription factors family was tested in tobacco plants, which were segregated to obtain F2 plants and were then subjected to water stress (drought) conditions to evaluate their function.

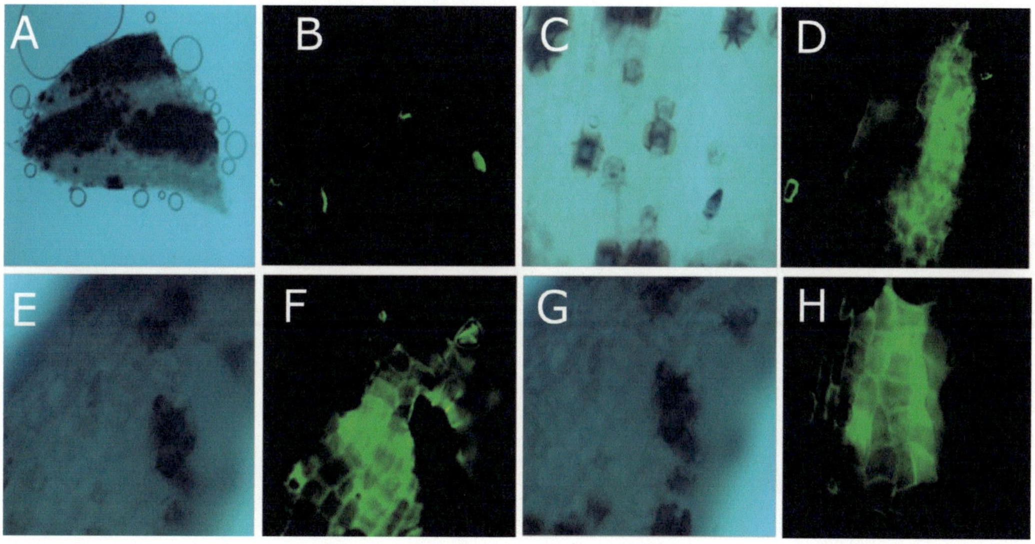

Figure 7. GFP fluorescence of different plant leaves of sugar cane var. MEX69290. (A) Segment of wild leaf in visible light. (B) Wild leaf segment with emission at 509 nm. (C, E and G) Transgenic plants 1, 2 and 3 in visible light. (D, F and H) Transgenic plants 1, 2 and 3 with emission at 509 nm.

7. Conclusions

Climate change affects farmers economically, causing drought floods, which affect the productivity of the plant. Biotechnology is an alternative to reduce the impact of climate change on plants. In recent years there has been a continuing need to provide commercial clones of resistance to pests and long-lasting diseases in combination with superior agronomic performance. This led to considerable research in different areas of biotechnology including: micropropagation, transcriptomics and genetic transformation.

These areas of biotechnology together are a key tool in the pursuit of genetically enhanced plants that resist climate change.

Abbreviations

BAC	Bacterial artificial chromosome
EST	Expressed sequence tag
NGS	Next generation sequencing
GO	Gene Ontology
ABA	Abscisic acid
LEA	Late embryogenesis abundant
NAC	NAM, ATAF, and CUC
MYB	Myeloblastosis
HSF	Heat shock factor
ZF	Zinc Finger
TF	Transcription factor
ORF	Open reading frame
aa	Amino acids
DEG	Differentially expressed genes
HMM	Hidden Markov Model
TMM	Trimmed mean of M values
DIR	Dirigent
nt	Nucleotide
H_2O_2	Hydrogen peroxide
NaCl	Sodium chloride

PEG	Polyethylene glycol
CA	Constitutive activity
GFP	Green fluorescent protein

Author details

Evelyn Arlette Carrillo Bermejo[1], Miguel Angel Herrera Alamillo[1], Samuel David Gamboa Tuz[1], Miguel Angel Keb Llanes[1], Enrique Castaño de la Serna[2], Manuel L. Robert[1] and Luis Carlos Rodríguez Zapata[1]*

*Address all correspondence to: lcrz@cicy.mx

1 Biotechnology Unit, Yucatan Scientific Research Center, Yucatan, Mexico

2 Unit of Biochemistry and Molecular Biology of Plants, Center for Scientific Research of Yucatan, Yucatan, Mexico

References

[1] Nelsona G, Valinb H, Sandsc R, Havlíkb P, Ahammadd H, Derynge D, et al. Climate change effects on agriculture: Economic responses to biophysical shocks. PNAS. 2014;**111**:3274-3279. DOI: 10.1073/pnas.1222465110

[2] Jahangir GZ, Nasir IA. Various hormonal supplementations activate sugarcane regeneration in vitro. Journal of Agricultural Science. 2010;**2**:231-237. DOI: 10.5539/jas.v2n4p231

[3] FAOSTAT. Sugarcane Production. Rome, Italy: Food and Agriculture Organization; 2014 [Internet]. Available from: http://faostat.fao.org/site/567/DesktopDefault.asp [Accessed: 21-02-2017]

[4] Sengar K. Developing an efficient protocol through tissue culture techniques for sugarcane micropropagation. BioInfoBank Library Acta. 2010;**18**:56

[5] Agarwal PK, Agarwal P, Reddy MK, Sopory SK. Role of DREB transcription factors in abiotic and biotic stress tolerance in plants. Plant Cell Reports. 2006;**25**:1263-1274. DOI: 10.1007/s00299-006-0204-8

[6] Burke EJ, Brown SJ, Christidis N. Modelling the recent evolution of global drought and projections for the twenty-first century with the Hadley Centre climate model. Journal of Hydrometeorology. 2006;**7**:1113-1125

[7] Shao HB, Chu LY, Jaleel CA, Zhao CX. Water-deficit stress-induced anatomical changes in higher plants. Comptes Rendus Biologies. 2008;**33**:215-225

[8] Moore PH, Paterson AH, Tew T. Sugarcane: The crop, the plant, and domestication. In: Moore PH, Botha FC, editors. Sugarcane: Physiology, Biochemistry, and Functional Biology. Chichester: John Wiley & Sons, Inc.; 2013. pp. 411-435. DOI: 10.1002/ 9781118771280.ch1

[9] Kingston G. Benchmarking yield of sugarcane from estimates of crop water use. Proceedings of the Australian Society for Sugar Cane Technologists. 1994;**16**:201-209

[10] Robertson MJ, Inmam-Bamber NG, Muchow RC, Wood AW. Physiology and productivity of sugarcane with early and mid-season water deficit. Field Crops Research. 1999;**64**:211-227. DOI: 10.1016/S0378-4290(99)00042-8

[11] Ramesh P. Effect of different levels of drought during the formative phase on growth parameters and its relationship with dry matter accumulation in sugarcane. Journal of Agricultural Science. 2000;**185**:83-89. DOI: 10.1046/j.1439-037x.2000.00404.x

[12] Basnayake J, Jackson PAN, Inman-Bamber G, Lakshmanan P. Sugarcane for water-limited environments. Genetic variation in cane yield and sugar content in response to water stress. Journal of Experimental Botany. 2012;**63**:6023-6033. DOI: 10.1093/jxb/ers251

[13] Gentile A, Dias LI, Mattos RS, Ferreira TH, Menossi M. MicroRNAs and drought responses in sugarcane. Frontiers in Plant Science. 2015;**6**:58. DOI: 10.3389/fpls.2015.00058

[14] Moreira J, Goswami D, Zhao Y, editors. Solar Energy and Human Settlement. Bioenergy-successes and barriers. In: Proceedings of ISES Solar World Congress. Vols. I–V; 2017. pp. 38-45

[15] Walter A, Galdos M, Scarpare F, Seabra J, Leal M, Cunha M. Brazilian sugarcane ethanol: Developments so far and challenges for the future. Wiley Interdisciplinary Reviews: Energy and Environment. 2013;**3**:70-92. DOI: 10.1002/wene.87

[16] Wang WX, Vinocur B, Shoseyov O, Altman A. Biotechnology of plant osmotic stress tolerance and physiological and molecular considerations. Acta Horticulturae. 2001;**560**:285-292. DOI: 10.17660/ActaHortic.2001.560.54

[17] Hasanuzzaman M, Nahar K, Alam MM, Roychowdhury R, Fujita M. Physiological, biochemical, and molecular mechanisms of heat stress tolerance in plants. International Journal of Molecular Sciences. 2013;**14**:9643-9684. DOI: 10.3390/ijms14059643

[18] Bartels D, Sunkar R. Drought and salt tolerance in plants. Critical Reviews in Plant Sciences. 2005;**24**:23-58. DOI: 10.1080/07352680590910410

[19] Smit M, Singels A. The response of sugarcane canopy development to water stress. Field Crops Research. 2006;**98**:91-97. DOI: 10.1016/j.fcr.2005.12.009

[20] Da Graça J, Rodrigues F, Farias J, Oliveira MD, Hoffmann-Campo C, Zingaretti S. Physiological parameters in sugarcane cultivars submitted to water deficit. Brazilian Journal of Plant Physiology. 2010;**22**:189-197. DOI: 10.1590/S1677-04202010000300006

[21] Inman-Bamber N, Lakshmanan P, Park S. Sugarcane for water limited environments: Theoretical assessment of suitable traits. Field Crops Research. 2012;**134**:95-104. DOI: 10.1016/j.fcr.2012.05.004

[22] Hemaprabha G, Nagarajan R, Alarmelu S. Response of sugarcane genotypes to water deficit stress. Sugar Tech. 2004;**6**:165-168. DOI: 10.1007/BF02942718

[23] Machado R, Ribeiro R, Marchiori P, Machado D, Machado E, Landell M. Biometric and physiological responses to water deficit in sugarcane at different phenological stages. Pesquisa Agropecuária Brasileira. 2009;**44**:1575-1582

[24] Inman-Bamber N. Sugarcane water stress criteria for irrigation and drying off. Field Crops Research. 2004;**89**:107-122. DOI: 10.1016/j.fcr.2004.01.018

[25] Inman-Bamber N, Bonnett G, Spillman M, Hewitt M, Jackson J. Increasing sucrose accumulation in sugarcane by manipulating leaf extension and photosynthesis with irrigation. Australian Journal of Agricultural Research. 2008;**59**:13-26. DOI: 10.1071/AR07167

[26] Inman-Bamber N, Smith D. Water relations in sugarcane and response to water deficits. Field Crops Research. 2005;**92**:185-202. DOI: 10.1016/j.fcr.2005.01.023

[27] Du Y, Kawamitsu Y, Nose A, Hiyane S, Murayama S, Wasano K, et al. Effects of water stress on carbon exchange rate and activities of photosynthetic enzymes in leaves of sugarcane (*Saccharum* sp.). Australian Journal of Plant Physiology. 1996;**23**:719-726. DOI: 10.1071/PP9960719

[28] Endres L, Silva JV, Ferreira VM, Barbosa GVS. Photosynthesis and water relations in Brazilian sugarcane. The Open Agriculture Journal. 2010;**4**:31-37. DOI: 10.2174/1874331501004010031

[29] Medeiros DB, da Silva EC, Mansur Custodio Nogueira RJ, Teixeira MM, Buckeridge MS. Physiological limitations in two sugarcane varieties under water suppression and after recovering. Theoretical and Experimental Plant Physiology. 2013;**25**:213-222. DOI: 10.1590/S2197-00252013000300006

[30] Basnayake J, Jackson PA, Inman-Bamber NG, Lakshmanan P. Sugarcane for water-limited environments. Variation in stomatal conductance and its genetic correlation with crop productivity. Journal of Experimental Botany. 2015;**66**:3945-3958. DOI: 10.1093/jxb/erv194

[31] Lakshmanan P, Robinson N. Stress physiology: Abiotic stresses. In: Moore PH, Botha FC, editors. Sugarcane: Physiology, Biochemistry, and Functional Biology. Chichester: John Wiley & Sons, Inc.; 2014. pp. 411-434

[32] McCormick AJ, Cramer MD, Watt DA. Regulation of photosynthesis by sugars in sugarcane leaves. Journal of Plant Physiology. 2008;**165**:1817-1829. DOI: 10.1016/j.jplph.2008.01.008

[33] Goldschmidt EE, Huber SC. Regulation of photosynthesis by endproduct accumulation in leaves of plants storing starch, sucrose, and hexose sugars. Plant Physiology. 1992;**99**:1443-1448. DOI: 10.1104/pp.99.4.1443

[34] Delorge I, Janiak M, Carpentier S, Van Dijck P. Fine tuning of trehalose biosynthesis and hydrolysis as novel tools for the generation of abiotic stress tolerant plants. Frontiers in Plant Science. 2014;**5**:147. DOI: 10.3389/fpls.2014.00147

[35] Sales CRG, Ribeiro RV, Machado DFSP, Machado RS, Dovis VL, Lagôa AMMA. Gas exchange and carbohydrate balance in sugarcane plants under root stressful conditions. Bragantia. 2012;**71**:319-327. DOI: 10.1590/S0006-87052012000300001

[36] Keating BA, Wilson JR. Intensive Sugarcane Production: Meeting the Challenge beyond 2000. Wallingford: CAB International; 1997

[37] Bakker H. Sugar Cane Cultivation and Management. New York: Kluwer Academic/ Plenum Publishers; 1999

[38] Ferreira THS, Tsunada MS, Bassi D, Araújo P, Mattiello L, Guidelli GV, Righetto GL, Goncalves VR, Lakshmanan P, Menossi M. Sugarcane water stress tolerance mechanisms and its implications on developing biotechnology solutions. Frontiers in Plant Science. 2017;**8**:1077. DOI: 10.3389/fpls.2017.01077

[39] Gomathi R, Gururaja Rao PN, Chandran K, Selvi A. Adaptive responses of sugarcane to waterlogging stress: An over view. Sugar Tech [Internet]. Springer India. 2015;**17**:325-338. Available from: http://dx.doi.org/10.1007/s12355-014-0319-0 [Accessed: 23-06-2017]

[40] Avivi S, Soeparjono S, Arieza Ramadhan R. Physiological characters of sugarcane after flooding stress. Agriculture and Agricultural Science Procedia [Internet]. Elsevier Srl. 2016;**9**:31-39. Available from: http://dx.doi.org/10.1016/j.aaspro.2016.02.119 [Accessed: 07-03-2017]

[41] Rojas-Martínez L, Visser RGF, de Klerk GJ. The hyperhydricity syndrome: Waterlogging of plant tissues as a major cause. Propagation of Ornamental Plants. 2010;**10**:169-175

[42] Dewir YH, Insoliya Y, Chakrabarty D, Paek KY. Biochemical and physiological aspects of hyperhydricity in liquid culture system. In: Paek KY, editor. Prod. Biomass Bioact. Compd. Using Bioreact. Technol. Netherlands: Springer; 2014. pp. 693-709

[43] Lyam PT, Musa ML, Jamaleddine ZO, Okere UA, Odofin WT. The potential of temporary immersion bioreactors (TIBs) in meeting crop production demand in Nigeria. Journal of Biology and Life Science. 2012;**3**:66-86

[44] Snyman SJ, Nkwanyana PD, Watt MP. Alleviation of hyperhydricity of sugarcane plantlets produced in RITA vessels and genotypic and phenotypic characterization of acclimated plants. South African Journal of Botany. [Internet]. SAAB. 2011;**77**:685-692. Available from: http://dx.doi.org/10.1016/j.sajb.2011.03.004 [Accessed: 09-05-2017]

[45] Tesfa M. In vitro shoot multiplication of elite sugarcane (*Saccharum officinarum* L.) genotypes using liquid shake culture system. Journal of Biology, Agriculture and Healthcare. 2016;**6**:35-40. DOI: 10.1590/S0100-204X2009001200003

[46] Arencibia AD, Bernal A, Yang L, Cortegaza L, Carmona ER, Pérez A, et al. New role of phenylpropanoid compounds during sugarcane micropropagation in Temporary Immersion Bioreactors (TIBs). Plant Science. 2008;**175**:487-496

[47] Bernal A, MacHado P, Cortegaza L, Carmona ER, Rivero O, Zayas CM, et al. Priming and biopriming integrated into the sugarcane micropropagation technology by Temporary Immersion Bioreactors (TIBS). Sugar Tech. 2008;**10**:42-47

[48] Silva M, Cabral E, Mota G, Willadino L, Camara T. In vitro propagation in Temporary Immersion System of sugarcane plants variety "RB 872552" derived from somatic embryos. Biotecnología Vegetal. 2015;**15**:187-191

[49] Li M, Liang Z, Zeng Y, Jing Y, Wu K, Liang J, Wang L. De novo analysis of transcriptome reveals genes associated with leaf abscission in sugarcane (*Saccharum officinarum* L.). BMC Genomics. 2016;**17**(1):195. DOI: 10.1186/s12864-016-2552-2

[50] Hoang NV, Furtado A, O'Keeffe AJ, Botha FC, Henry RJ. Association of gene expression with biomass content and composition in sugarcane. PLoS One. 2017;**12**(8):1-31. DOI: 10.1371/journal.pone.0183417

[51] Belesini AA, Carvalho FMS, Telles BR, Castro GM, Giachetto PF, Vantini JS, Carlin SD, Cazetta JO, Pinheiro DG, Ferro MIT. De novo transcriptome assembly of sugarcane leaves submitted to prolonged water-deficit stress. Genetics and Molecular Research: GMR. 2017;**16**(2):1-20. DOI: 10.4238/gmr16028845

[52] Pereira-Santana A, Alvarado-Robledo EJ, Zamora-Briseño JA, Ayala-Sumuano JT, Gonzalez Mendoza VM, Espadas-Gil F, et al. Transcriptional profiling of sugarcane leaves and roots under progressive osmotic stress reveals a regulated coordination of gene expression in a spatiotemporal manner. PLoS One. 2017;**12**(12):1-25. DOI: 10.1371/journal.pone.0189271

[53] Gu Z, Eils R, Schlesner M. Complex heatmaps reveal patterns and correlations in multidimensional genomic data. Bioinformatics. 2016;**32**(18):2847-2849. DOI: 10.1093/bioinformatics/btw313

[54] R Development Core Team. R: A Language and Environment for Statistical Computing. Vienna, Austria [Internet]; 2017. Available from: https://www.r-project.org/ [Accessed: 10-08-2017]

[55] Finn RD, Coggill P, Eberhardt RY, Eddy SR, Mistry J, Mitchell AL, Bateman A. The Pfam protein families database: Towards a more sustainable future. Nucleic Acids Research. 2016;**44**(D1):D279-D285. DOI: 10.1093/nar/gkv1344

[56] Goodstein DM, Shu S, Howson R, Neupane R, Hayes RD, Fazo J, Rokhsar DS. Phytozome: A comparative platform for green plant genomics. Nucleic Acids Research. 2012;**40**(D1):D1178. DOI: 10.1093/nar/gkr944

[57] Ralph S, Park JY, Bohlmann J, Mansfield SD. Dirigent proteins in conifer defense: Gene discovery, phylogeny, and differential wound- and insect-induced expression of a family of DIR and DIR-like genes in spruce (*Picea* spp.). Plant Molecular Biology. 2006;**60**(1):21. DOI: 10.1007/s11103-005-2226-y

[58] Zhu L, Zhang X, Tu L, Zeng F, Nie Y, Guo X. Isolation and characterization of two novel dirigent-like genes highly induced in cotton (*Gossypium barbadense* and *G. hirsutum*) after infection by *Verticillium dahliae*. Journal of Plant Pathology. 2007;**89**:41-45

[59] Wu R, Wang L, Wang Z, Shang H, Liu X, Zhu Y, Deng X. Cloning and expression analysis of a dirigent protein gene from the resurrection plant *Boea hygrometrica*. Progress in Natural Science. 2009;**19**(3):347-352. DOI: 10.1016/j.pnsc.2008.07.010

[60] Jin-long G, Li-ping X, Jing-ping F, Ya-chun S, Hua-ying F, You-xiong Q, Jing-sheng X. A novel dirigent protein gene with highly stem-specific expression from sugarcane, response to drought, salt and oxidative stresses. Plant Cell Reports. 2012;**31**(10):1801-1812. DOI: 10.1007/s00299-012-1293-1

[61] Nobile PM, Bottcher A, Mayer JLS, Brito MS, dos Anjos IA, de Andrade Landell MG, Mazzafera P. Identification, classification and transcriptional profiles of dirigent domain-containing proteins in sugarcane. Molecular Genetics and Genomics. 2017;**292**(6):1323-1340. DOI: 10.1007/s00438-017-1349-6

[62] Anderson DJ, Birch RG. Minimal handling and super-binary vectors facilitate efficient, Agrobacterium-mediated, transformation of sugarcane (*Saccharum* spp. hybrid). Tropical Plant Biology. 2012;**5**:183-192. DOI: 10.1007/s12042-012-9101-1

[63] Niu J-Q, Wang A-Q, Huang J-L, Yang L-T, Li Y-R. Isolation, characterization and promoter analysis of cell wall invertase gene SoCIN1 from sugarcane (*Saccharum* spp.). Sugar Tech. 2014;**17**(1):65-76. DOI: 10.1007/s12355-014-0348-8

[64] Yogesh T, Maria G, Fredy A. Comparison of direct and indirect embryogenesis protocols, biolistic gene transfer and selection parameters for efficient genetic transformation of sugarcane. Plant Cell, Tissue and Organ Culture (PCTOC). 2012;**111**:131-141. DOI: 10.1007/s11240-012-0177-y

[65] Zale J, Jung JH, Kim JY, Pathak B, Karan R, Liu H, Chen X, Wu H, Candreva J, Zhai Z, Shanklin J, Altpeter F. Metabolic engineering of sugarcane to accumulate energy-dense triacylglycerols in vegetative biomass. Plant Biotechnology Journal. 2016;**14**:661-669

[66] Arencibia AD, Carmona ER. Sugarcane (*Saccharum* spp.). In: Wang K, editor. Agrobacterium Protocols. 2nd ed. Totowa, NJ: Humana Press; 2006. pp. 227-235. DOI: 10.1385/1-59745-131-2:227

[67] Manickavasagam M, Ganapathi A, Anbazhagan VR, Sudhakar B, Selvaraj N, Vasudevan A, Kasthurirengan S. Agrobacterium-mediated genetic transformation and development of herbicide-resistant sugarcane (*Saccharum* species hybrids) using axillary buds. Plant Cell Reports. 2004;**23**:134-143. DOI: 10.1007/s00299-004-0794-y

[68] Reis RR, da Cunha BADB, Martins PK, Martins MTB, Alekcevetch JC, Chalfun-Júnior A, et al. Induced over-expression of AtDREB2A CA improves drought tolerance in sugarcane. Plant Science. 2014;**221**:59-68. DOI: 10.1016/j.plantsci.2014.02.003

Section 3

Plant Resposes to Climatic Changes

Plant Metabolomics in a Changing World: Metabolite Responses to Abiotic Stress Combinations

Tiago F. Jorge and Carla António

Additional information is available at the end of the chapter

http://dx.doi.org/10.5772/intechopen.71769

Abstract

Climate change constitutes a real threat to the global landscape. Current climate models predict an increased occurrence of coastal floods associated to sea level rise and long-term droughts associated to changes in the intra- and inter-year rainfall variability. Under natural environmental conditions, plants are routinely exposed to abiotic stresses, and must develop different strategies to cope with this multitude of climate change factors. Mass spectrometry (MS)-based plant metabolomics approaches are finding an increasing number of applications to investigate the molecular and biochemical mechanisms that underlie plant responses to changing environments. These studies provide a promising basis for facilitating our understanding of the plant's flexibility to reconfigure central metabolic pathways (i.e., carbon, nitrogen and energy metabolism) as well as the degree by which plants tolerate and/or are susceptible to a climate change scenario. In this chapter, we will provide an update on the recent MS-based metabolomics strategies to study plant responses to drought, salt and heat stress as well as combinations thereof. We will describe how these stresses activate and coordinate several different signalling pathways, for example, through the synthesis of osmolytes.

Keywords: plant metabolomics, drought stress, salinity stress, heat stress, stress combination, climate change, mass spectrometry

1. Introduction

Climate change can be defined as a statistically significant variation in the weather pattern or in its variability during a long-term period [1]. The causes of climate change have been mainly associated to (i) internal environmental processes and (ii) anthropogenic activities that lead to changes in the chemical composition of the atmosphere [1]. Natural climate variability itself is not enough to explain the unforeseen weather changes in the last decades. In fact, since the industrial revolution that human-kind activities (e.g., fossil fuel burning) have also contributed to the release of significant amounts of greenhouse gases (GHGs) namely CO_2, CH_4, N_2O as well as fluorinated gases to the atmosphere [1]. Indeed, climate change assessments have reported that the global atmospheric CO_2 concentration has increased from 270 to 401 $\mu L\ L^{-1}$ since the industrial revolution, and consequently, the average global temperatures to rise by 0.85°C. Moreover, global warming has been reported to be highly correlated with ocean thermal expansion and loss of glacier mass, which ultimately reflected the observed global mean sea level rise of 0.19 ± 0.02 m over the period 1901–2010 [2]. By the end of the twenty-first century, unmatched climate changes are envisaged with CO_2 concentrations of at least 700 $\mu L\ L^{-1}$ and global temperatures are expected to rise at least 4°C. Consequently, higher surface temperatures, longer and frequent heat waves and intense extreme precipitation events are very likely to occur in many regions around the globe. The consequences from climate change cannot be totally avoided, but without additional mitigation efforts beyond those already in place today, warming by the end of the twenty-first century will lead to very high risk of severe and irreversible impacts globally [2].

Extreme climate change events expose plants to stressful environmental conditions that are outside of their physiological limits, and beyond the range by which they are already adapted [3]. Studies aiming at assessing the impact of climate change in plant ecosystems revealed that plant community responses occur at three sequential levels in which (i) climate change immediately impacts plant individuals at the morpho-physiological level, (ii) the community response is affected because of demographic changes in species abundances and (iii) the mortality or loss of species leads to their replacement by novel species within the community [4–6]. Although some studies have contributed to a better understanding of plant ecosystem responses to climate change, this research field is still emerging. A comprehensive discussion on this topic falls outside the scope of this chapter, and detailed information can be found elsewhere [4–13].

Responses by individual plant species to climate change have been indirectly studied through the assessment of the strategies and mechanisms by which they cope with adverse environmental conditions, that is, abiotic stresses. Abiotic stresses in plants comprise a multitude of environmental factors such as water (drought, flooding and submergence), temperature (high and low), light (high and low), radiation (UV-B and UV-A), salinity and nutrients, heavy metals, among others. These environmental (stress)factors negatively affect plant growth and development, and trigger a series of high-complex adaptive responses initiated by stress perception, signal transduction and the activation of many stress-related genes and metabolites [14, 15]. However, under natural environmental conditions, plants are routinely exposed to a combination of different abiotic stresses, and therefore, must develop different strategies to cope with a multitude of environmental factors. The latter gains more relevance under climate change scenarios, and therefore, there has been an increasing interest in understanding the molecular and biochemical mechanisms that underlie plant responses to abiotic stress combinations [16, 17].

Many studies, at both physiological and biochemical levels, have been performed to study plant responses to different stress combinations namely drought, salt, extreme temperatures and biotic stresses. Interestingly, these studies demonstrated that a plant response to a combined stress is unique, and should not be regarded as the sum of the responses from each applied stress alone. Additionally, when different stresses are combined, they might require synergistic or antagonistic responses that are largely controlled by, sometimes, opposing signalling pathways [16, 17]. In this chapter, we will provide an update on recent studies of plant responses to drought, salt and heat stress as well as combinations thereof. We will describe how these abiotic stress combinations activate and coordinate several different signalling pathways, for example, through the synthesis of osmolytes, in order to ensure plant survival.

2. Metabolomics—a key *omics* tool to study plant responses to abiotic stress

Over the past decade, plant metabolomics has undoubtedly become a powerful research tool to study the biochemical mechanisms underlying plant growth and development in the context of plant metabolite responses to abiotic stress, particularly drought, flooding, salinity and extreme temperatures (heat and cold). In fact, metabolomics itself, together with the other *omics* technologies (genomics, transcriptomics and proteomics) has accelerated our understanding of the complex molecular interactions in biological systems [18–24] (**Figure 1**). Moreover, unlike other *omics* tools, metabolomics has the advantage of not being dependent on the availability of organism-specific genome information for data analysis [25–27]. The main goal of plant metabolomics is to provide a non-biased characterisation of the total metabolite pool of a plant tissue in response to its environment. This metabolite pool includes a wide range of metabolites with diverse physical properties, from ionic inorganic compounds to biochemically derived hydrophilic carbohydrates, organic and amino acids, and a range of hydrophobic lipid-related compounds. Indeed, it is estimated that more than 200,000 different primary and secondary metabolites exist in the plant kingdom over a large dynamic range in concentrations that can vary from femtomolar to millimolar [28]. While, primary metabolites are fundamental for plant growth and development, being highly conserved in their molecular structures and abundances throughout the plant kingdom, secondary metabolites help plants communicating with the environment and widely differ across species. Due to such metabolite diversity, current plant metabolomics studies often combine multiple analytical tools in an effort to acquire more comprehensive metabolite coverage from a complex biological plant sample. One powerful analytical tool is nuclear magnetic resonance (NMR); however, due

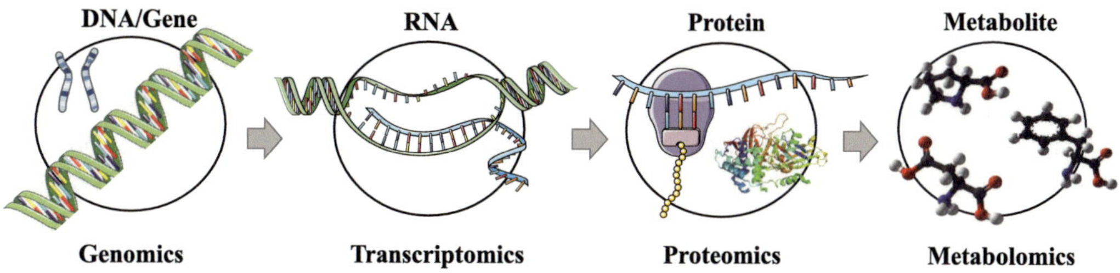

Figure 1. *Omics* technologies have accelerated our understanding of the complex molecular interactions in biological systems.

to its poor sensitivity and poor dynamic range relative to mass spectrometry (MS) [29, 30], MS-based analytical tools are the most widely used in plant metabolomics. Among them, powerful chromatographic techniques such as liquid chromatography-mass spectrometry (LC-MS) and gas chromatography-mass spectrometry (GC-MS) have been extensively used to obtain comprehensive information of the plant metabolome in a wide range of plant species [24, 31]. Regardless the analytical platform of choice, great attention must be paid to the experimental design. In plant metabolomics, an adequate and well-studied experimental design should address different environmental and experimental variables such as (i) plant tissue harvest, (ii) metabolic quenching and (iii) metabolite extraction methods. In addition, randomisation procedures throughout all the experimental workflow should be taken into account to minimise potential sources of experimental errors [32, 33]. A detailed discussion of sample preparation workflows and MS-based analytical platforms typically used in plant metabolomics experiments can be found elsewhere [24, 34].

3. Plant metabolite responses to individual abiotic stresses

Metabolite responses to individual abiotic stresses such as drought, salinity or heat have been widely studied, and comprehensive reviews on this topic can be found in the literature [24, 31]. In this section, we describe recent applications of MS-based metabolomics approaches to study plant responses to individual abiotic stresses, namely drought, salt and heat stress, highlighting the identification of stress-responsive metabolites that ultimately contribute for the development of plants with enhanced abiotic stress-tolerance.

3.1. Metabolite responses to drought stress

Drought is a well-studied abiotic stress, and one major limiting factor in agriculture worldwide [35–37]. This stress condition leads to huge reductions in crop yields mainly derived from a series of morpho-physiological changes such as reduction in shoot growth [38], decreases in photosynthesis and transpiration rates as a direct consequence of abscisic acid (ABA)-mediated leaf stomata closure [36, 37] as well as changes in signalling pathways [36] and transcriptional and posttranscriptional regulation of several stress-related genes [39, 40]. In addition, plant metabolism is also readjusted under drought stress conditions through the accumulation of osmolytes or compatible solutes [41, 42]. These small molecules can accumulate at high concentrations in the cell without inhibiting cellular metabolism, and comprise, for example, soluble sugars and sugar alcohols such as glucose, sucrose and mannitol; the raffinose family oligosaccharides (RFOs) such as raffinose, stachyose and verbascose, amino acids and polyamines. Because of this osmolyte accumulation, a decrease in the osmotic potential of the cell is observed and the turgor pressure is maintained as the cell uptakes water, thereby help in stabilising membranes, enzymes and proteins, or maintaining cell turgor by osmotic adjustment. In addition, osmolyte accumulation also confers protection against oxidative damage by decreasing the levels of reactive oxygen species (ROS), which in turn, helps re-establish cellular redox balance. Consequently, osmotic adjustment is commonly recognised as an effective factor of drought tolerance in several plants to enable water uptake and the maintenance of plant metabolic activity, hence, growth and productivity as the water potential decreases [36, 37]. Drought stress has been widely reported to increase the production of ROS in different cellular compartments (i.e., oxidative stress) [43]. However, this oxidative stress has shown to lead to the formation of specific peptides that might counterbalance the accumulation of ROS upon abiotic stress conditions [44]. Nevertheless, ROS species are known to interact with proteins, lipids and DNA during abiotic stress episodes, and thus impair the normal function of cells [45–47].

Comprehensive omics studies have been reported to investigate plant responses to drought stress [42, 48–50]. An interesting study developed by Gechev and collaborators [51] addressed the molecular mechanisms of desiccation in *Haberlea rhodopensis* through transcriptomics and metabolomics approaches. The complementary use of GC-TOF-MS and LC-MS metabolite analyses revealed significant accumulation in the levels of the soluble sugars sucrose and maltose as wells as of the RFOs stachyose and verbascose in *H. rhodopensis* plants upon dehydration. Furthermore, and together with transcriptomics, these results were associated to *H. rhodopensis* ability to survive under dehydration conditions [51].

A similar comprehensive metabolomics approach was applied to study the resurrection plant *Selaginella lepidophylla* [52]. Metabolite profiles from ultra-high-performance liquid chromatography-tandem mass spectrometry (UHPLC-MS/MS) and GC-MS analysis revealed an accumulation of metabolites involved in the glycolytic pathway (glucose-6-phosphate, fructose-6-phosphate and pyruvate) as well as in the TCA cycle (2-oxoglutarate, succinate, fumarate and oxaloacetate) in hydrated *S. lepidophylla* plants. In parallel, the accumulation of the sugar alcohols sorbitol, myo-inositol and mannitol was related to the desiccation mechanisms developed by resurrection plants, which involve water uptake or loss during the rehydration/dehydration cycle [52].The moderate long-term drought stress effects was investigated in 21 rice cultivars (*Oryza sativa* L. ssp. indica and japonica) through physiological, gene expression and GC-TOF-MS metabolite profiling analysis [53]. Overall, this comprehensive study revealed that in rice, drought conditions induce an accumulation of spermine, thereby leading to a coordinated adjustment of polyamine metabolism which is in agreement with an osmoprotectant role of this metabolite under drought stress [53].

Meyer and co-workers [54] analysed at transcriptional, physiological and metabolite levels the responses to soil drying of the perennial C4 grass and biofuel crop, *Panicum virgatum* L. (switchgrass). In this study, genes associated with C4 photosynthesis were down-regulated during drought, while C4 metabolic intermediates have shown to accumulate. GC-TOF-MS data revealed that the abundance of 13 primary metabolites was significantly affected by the drought treatment and that most of these compounds also accumulated amino acids (>32-fold), monosaccharides (>14-fold) and organic acids (>four-fold) [54]).

GC-TOF-MS metabolite profiling in the leaves and roots of two barley (*Hordeum vulgare* L.) genotypes, with contrasting drought tolerance, revealed approximately 100 drought stress-responsive metabolites with amino acids being the most affected metabolite class. Together with proteomics data, this study indicated that the proteins and metabolites that have shown to accumulate in the susceptible variety also revealed elevated constitutive accumulation levels in the drought-resistant line. Moreover, the accumulation of several carbohydrates was affected in tissues of both genotypes subjected to drought [55].

In sunflower (*Helianthus annuus* L.), molecular mechanisms to drought tolerance were recently addressed through the characterisation and integration of transcriptional and metabolic data. GC-TOF-MS analysis allowed detecting 54 primary metabolites, including different amino acids, organic acids, sugars and sugar alcohols. This analysis revealed that most of the amino acids showed lower levels under drought with exception to proline, tyramine, glycine, malonate and γ-aminobutyrate (GABA), which accumulated upon drought conditions. On the other hand, glycolysis and tricarboxylic acid cycle (TCA) metabolites as well as all the detected carbohydrates showed higher levels under drought conditions. Overall, these results indicated the putative role of these metabolites during stress response in sunflower [56].

Another interesting study investigated osmoadaptation to drought stress in leaves and roots of cowpea (*Vigna unguiculata* L. Walp.) through analysis of photosynthetic traits, water homoeostasis, inorganic ions and primary and secondary metabolites. In this study, physiological and metabolite changes were shown to develop in parallel while drought/recovery responses revealed a progressive acclimation of the cowpea plant to stress. GC-TOF-MS analysis and subsequent multifactorial analyses indicated allocation of high quantities of amino acids, sugars and proanthocyanidins into roots, which were linked to their role in growth and initial stress perception. From the 88 metabolites detected, proline, galactinol and a quercetin derivative, were those that most responded to drought. In addition, these metabolites accumulated differently in roots, but similarly in leaves, suggesting a more conservative strategy to cope with drought in the aerial parts of cowpea plants [57].

3.2. Metabolite responses to salt stress

Soil salinity significantly reduces crop yields, being considered a global problem that affects approximately 20% of irrigated land [58]. The effects of salt stress in plants occur in two different sequential stages. In a first stage, the plant perceives osmotic stress, which reduces the plant's ability to uptake water, decreases cell turgor and leads to the accumulation of ROS in the cells. Subsequently, a second stage is initiated by an over accumulation of Na^+ and Cl^- ions that severely affect key plant physiological processes including photosynthesis, plasma membrane stability and cellular metabolism [59]. Consequently, plant growth and fertility are reduced, and premature senescence occurs [59, 60]. Plant susceptibility or tolerance to salt stress strongly depends on the mechanisms used by the plant to detoxify ROS species within the cells and exclude Na^+ ions from the roots or to compartmentalise these ions in the vacuoles [59, 61]. To cope with salt stress, plants adjust their metabolic status, and although this metabolic adjustment widely differs among salt-tolerant species, several common salt-stress metabolite responses are found within the plant kingdom [62, 63].

According to their salt tolerance, plants are usually divided in glycophytes (salt-sensitive) and halophytes (salt-tolerant). For glycophytic plants, there is an increasing evidence that amino acids, sugars, sugar alcohols and tricarboxylic acid (TCA)-cycle intermediates, form the core of metabolite adjustments to salinity stress [24, 31, 62]. On the other hand, for halophytic or extremophile plants, the pre-accumulation and differential response of osmoprotectant metabolites varies among plant species. Interestingly, a comparative study using both salt-sensitive and salt-tolerant Lotus species has demonstrated that around 50% of all metabolites have a comparable response to salinity [64]. A similar scenario was observed for *Arabidopsis thaliana* (salt-sensitive) and its distant relative *Thellungiella halophila* (salt-tolerant), both accumulating proline and soluble sugars (fructose, glucose, sucrose and raffinose) [65].

Among crops, an interesting study on barley (*Hordeum vulgare* L.) cultivars that differed in salt-stress tolerance were analysed for their metabolite response to long-term salt stress [66]. While the most tolerant cultivar Sahara showed elevated levels of hexose phosphates and TCA cycle intermediates, the levels of these metabolites remained unaffected during salinity stress in the less-tolerant cultivar Clipper [66]. In another study, wild barley showed to be more salt-tolerant than cultivated barley by accumulating more carbohydrates (sucrose, trehalose and raffinose) and proline in its roots than its cultivated counterpart, therefore demonstrating an improved ability to regulate osmotic stress [67]. Rice represents one of the most-sensitive cereal crops; however, a GC-TOF-MS analysis revealed lower levels of TCA cycle intermediates and other organic acids in the roots of more-tolerant rice cultivars than in those more sensitive. On the other hand, accumulation of amino acids was detected in the salt-tolerant rice cultivars [68].

A modern metabolomics approach based on two complementary highly sensitive approaches, namely GC- and LC-coupled to a triple quadrupole mass spectrometer (GC-QqQ-MS and LC-QqQ-MS), was applied for the quantitative profiling of a wide range of metabolites from two chickpea (*Cicer arietinum* L.) cultivars with contrasting responses to salt stress. While the GC-QqQ-MS metabolite profiling approach allowed to quantitatively analyse 48 primary metabolites, ranging from sugars and sugar phosphates to organic acids, the LC-QqQ-MS approach allowed to quantitatively measure 28 biogenic amines and amino acids. Furthermore, this complementary approach indicated that the metabolic differences between the two contrasting cultivars relied on metabolites involved in carbon metabolism, TCA cycle as well as amino acid metabolism [69]. A better elucidation of the physiological and biochemical processes of a salt-resistant maize (*Zea mays* L.) hybrid was achieved with GC-TOF-MS metabolite profiling analysis. By comparing a salt-sensitive and a salt-resistant maize hybrid, Richter and co-workers [70] could observe the accumulation of neutral sugars (glucose, fructose and sucrose) in the leaves of the salt-sensitive hybrid and regard these metabolites accumulation as a salt-resistance adaptation. In addition, both hybrids showed a strong decrease in the levels of TCA cycle intermediates [70].

Actinorhizal plants are a group of perennial dicotyledonous angiosperms. These plants are not only of economic importance (production of wood and derivatives), but are also highly resilient to extreme environments. *Casuarina glauca*, the model actinorhizal plant, is characterised by its ability to establish symbiosis with nitrogen-fixing *Frankia* bacteria and can thrive under extreme salinity conditions [71, 72]. However, until now, only few reports investigating the mechanisms underlying salt stress tolerance in actinorhizal plants are available, and most of these studies are not broad enough to grasp the complexity of the response. To better understand *C. glauca* ability to tolerate high levels of salinity, Jorge and collaborators [74] have pioneered a metabolomics study to investigate the impact of salt stress in *C. glauca* nodulated (NOD+) and non-nodulated (KNO_3+) plants subjected to different salinity levels (0 control, 200, 400 and 600 mM [NaCl]) [73]. GC-TOF-MS metabolite profiling data revealed major metabolite divergences in amino acid metabolism in both plant groups (NOD+ and KNO_3+).

Subsequent multivariate statistical analysis allowed concluding that modifications in the metabolite levels of neutral sugars, proline and ornithine revealed to be central in conferring tolerance to high levels of salinity in *C. glauca*. Furthermore, the same study also concluded that the main differences observed in the metabolite pool between NOD+ and KNO_3+ plants not only rely on the impact of the salt stress itself [73], but also on the disruption of the symbiotic activity of *C. glauca* NOD+ plants at early salt stress exposure (i.e., 200 mM [NaCl]) [74].

3.3. Metabolite responses to heat stress

Heat stress is often defined as the rise in temperature beyond a threshold level (usually 10–15°C) above ambient temperature, for an enough period of time, to cause irreversible damage to plant growth and development. The impact of heat stress depends not only on the temperature intensity but also on its duration and rate of increase [75, 76].

When a plant perceives exposure to heat stress, a series of cellular and molecular responses are known to be initiated, such as increased fluidity of lipid membranes, inactivation of key enzymes in some organelles (chloroplasts and mitochondria) and protein denaturation and aggregation. The ability of some plants to grow, develop and give profit under these circumstances is defined as heat tolerance. In plants, the heat stress response (HSR) pathway has been extensively studied [77–79]; however, a more comprehensive understanding of this pathway remains unclear [76].

Heat tolerance has been widely reported in the literature as being mediated by the synthesis of stress-related proteins, also known as heat shock proteins (HSPs) [77, 80]. This class of proteins has shown to confer heat tolerance by reducing the impact of high temperatures in photosynthesis, in carbon assimilate partitioning, in water and nutrient use efficiency as well as in keeping membrane stability [81–83]. General plant cellular and molecular responses to heat stress have been thoroughly reviewed elsewhere [75, 76, 79, 84, 85].

Metabolomics studies on plants subjected to heat stress have reported the accumulation of osmolytes, namely soluble sugars, glycine-betaine and proline [86]. In addition, high temperatures have been reported to disrupt sugar metabolism and proline transport during male reproductive development in tomato (*Solanum lycopersicum* L.) [87].

Du and co-workers [88] applied a GC-MS metabolite profiling approach to identify metabolites associated with differential heat tolerance between two grass species, namely C4 bermudagrass and C3 Kentucky bluegrass [88]. In both grass species, 36 heat stress-responsive metabolites were identified, ranging from organic and amino acids to sugars and sugar alcohols. However, most of these metabolites showed higher accumulation in bermudagrass when compared with Kentucky bluegrass. Among the differentially accumulated metabolites, this study reported seven sugars (sucrose, fructose, galactose, floridoside, melibiose, maltose and xylose), a sugar alcohol (inositol), six organic acids (malic acid, citric acid, threonic acid, galacturonic acid, isocitric acid and methyl malonic acid) and nine amino acids (asparagine, alanine, valine, threonine, GABA, isoleucine, glycine, lysine and methionine) [88].

Using a similar GC-MS metabolic profiling approach, Li and co-workers [89] investigated whether increased GABA levels could improve heat tolerance in cool-season creeping bentgrass

(*Agrostis Stolonifera* L.) [89]. Upon exogenous application of GABA, metabolite profiling data revealed an accumulation in the levels of six amino acids (glutamic acid, aspartic acid, alanine, threonine, serine and valine), five organic acids (aconitic acid, malic acid, succinic acid, oxalic acid and threonic acid), five sugars (sucrose, fructose, glucose, galactose and maltose) and two sugar alcohols (mannitol and myo-inositol). Together with physiological measurements, this study suggested that the GABA-induced heat tolerance in creeping bentgrass might result from three main factors (i) balance of photosynthesis and transpiration, (ii) improvement of the ascorbate-glutathione cycle and (ii) maintenance of osmotic adjustment. Furthermore, an increase in the levels of metabolites involved in the GABA shunt (glutamic acid, GABA and alanine) was suggested to act as an intermediate supplier to feed the TCA cycle during a long-term heat stress, thereby maintaining metabolic homeostasis [89].

4. Plant metabolite responses to abiotic stress combinations

Plant abiotic stress studies typically deal with the comparison of a few genotypes (tolerant versus sensitive species) grown under controlled conditions, followed by the analysis and identification of differential responses to the imposed stress. Yet, these conditions are unlikely to reproduce field conditions in which a range of abiotic stresses is likely to occur simultaneously. Abiotic stress combinations, such as those involving drought and salinity, salinity and heat as well as drought and extreme temperature or high light intensity are the most commonly reported stress combinations in field conditions [17, 90]. Pioneering abiotic stress combination studies, that involved drought and heat stress, were performed in tobacco (*Nicotiana tabacum* L.) and in the model plant *A. thaliana*. These studies revealed that the molecular responses to this stress combination are unique and should not be regarded as the sum of the responses from each individually applied stress [17, 91, 92]. Afterwards, significant studies have been performed to elucidate the plant molecular responses to several abiotic stress combinations that include drought, salt, extreme temperatures, heavy metals, UV-B, high light, ozone, CO_2, soil compaction and biotic stresses (e.g., pathogen attack) [17, 93]. Likewise, these studies also reported that each stress combination requires specific plant molecular responses. Among them, specific physiological responses as well as specific regulatory transcripts, proteins and metabolites were found for each stress combination under study. Having said this, plant responses to combined stresses require an orchestration of specific metabolic and signalling responses such as antioxidant mechanisms or the synthesis of osmolytes [90, 92, 94–98].

In 2006, Mittler [16] developed an intuitive diagram denominated "*Stress Matrix*" in which the result of a positive and/or negative interaction between two different stress combinations on plant growth, yield and physiological traits can be easily described [16]. Since then, this matrix has been updated several times [17, 93, 99] (**Figure 2**). According to **Figure 2**, most abiotic stress combination studies include drought or salinity as one of the main stress conditions. Stress combinations between drought and heat, salinity and heat, ozone and salinity, ozone and heat, nutrient stress and drought, nutrient stress and salinity (to name a few) were reported to have a higher negative impact on plant development than when each different stress component is applied individually. On the other hand, combinations of drought and ozone, high CO_2 with ozone, salt

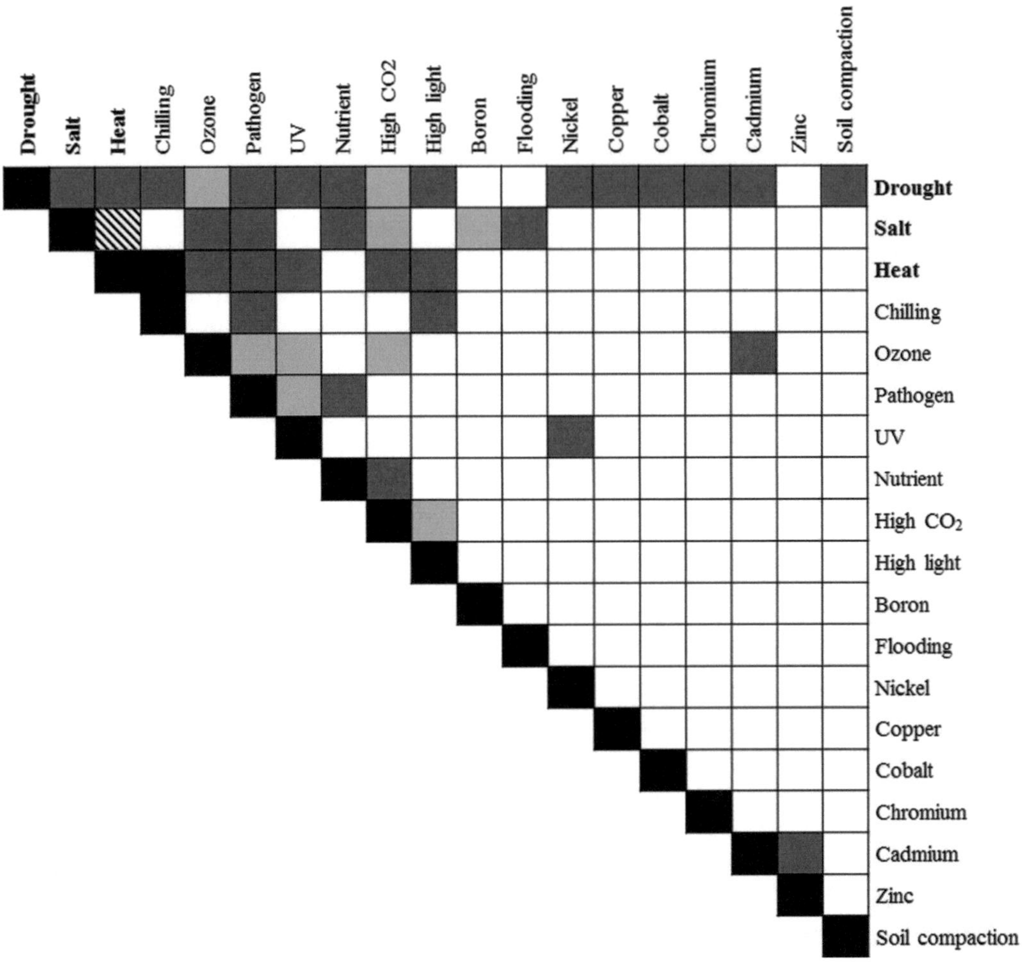

Figure 2. Intuitive "*Stress Matrix*" showing the result of a positive (light grey) and/or negative (dark grey) interaction between two different stress combinations on plant growth, yield and physiological traits. Striped-pattern square indicates a not well-studied species specific-interaction (might be positive and/or negative) (adapted from [16, 17, 97, 103]).

or high light were shown to have a favourable effect on plants as compared to when each different stress component is applied individually [17, 99]. Interestingly, the combination of salinity and heat stress has shown to provide both positive and negative interactions. These conflicting results suggest that the positive or negative effects of a stress combination could be dependent on the plant genotype, species and/or timing and intensity of the different stresses involved. Considering the increased number of heat waves and rising seawater levels expected for the next decades [2], the study of plant metabolite responses to salt and heat stress in a wide range of species is therefore predicted to become increasingly relevant in the current climate change context.

4.1. Metabolite responses to combined drought and heat stress

The effect of drought and heat stress on plant growth and development is currently the most well-studied abiotic stress combination [16, 17, 90], mainly because these two environmental-stress factors are the most representative in the field. In addition, they are the primary environmental stresses that determine the distribution and productivity of plants [91, 100]. Following the pioneering studies of the effects of combined drought and heat stress in tobacco and *A. thaliana* [91], many similar studies have been carried out in several other plant species and crops [16, 17, 90, 93, 101]. One interesting study is that of Obata and collaborators [102] who aimed at dissecting the metabolite responses induced by drought, heat and the combination of both stresses in 10 tropical maize hybrids. Through the integration of physiological and metabolomics data, this study identified promising metabolite marker candidates [102]. Under drought stress, GC-TOF-MS analysis of maize leaves revealed the accumulation of several amino acids (isoleucine, valine, threonine, 4-aminobutanoate, glycine and serine) as well as the accumulation of the sugar alcohol *myo*-inositol. On the other hand, when both drought and heat stress were combined, metabolite responses could be predicted from the sum of individual stresses as only a few specific responses could be observed [102].

Metabolite changes under this stress combination were also assessed in the fleshy herbaceous plant Purslane (*Portulaca oleracea* L.) [103]. In total, GC-TOF-MS analysis allowed detecting 37 primary metabolites. Of these, fructose, galactose and xylitol were only detected in control plants; alanine, sorbose, glucose and heptulose were only detected in drought stress-treated plants; glycine, threonine and asparagine were only detected in heat stress-treated plants, while isoleucine and phenylalanine were only found in combined stress-treated plants. On the other hand, propionic acid, gluconic acid, mannose and urea were detected in both individual and combined stress-treated plants. Overall, this study allowed to conclude that the main strategies adopted by purslane to survive drought, heat, and combined drought and heat stress, involves the accumulation of osmoprotectant metabolites and an increase in the antioxidative system [103].

The impact of combined drought and heat stress has also been evaluated in the crop plant soybean (*Glycine max* L.) through a comprehensive MS-based metabolomics approach comprising LC- and GC-MS analysis [104]. This approach allowed identifying 266 putative metabolites, including primary and secondary metabolites. Subsequent statistical analysis revealed that combined drought and heat stress induced a differentially accumulation of several metabolites in soybean leaves, such as sugars, amino acids and lipids. Moreover, individual stresses (i.e., drought or heat) affected key metabolites involved in different pathways such as glycolysis, TCA cycle, the pentose phosphate pathway and starch biosynthesis. That said, this study demonstrated that sugar and nitrogen metabolism are essential in soybean to cope with drought and heat stress conditions [104].

4.2. Metabolite responses to combined drought and salt stress

With increasing earth surface temperatures, it is very likely that regions of high surface salinity, where evaporation dominates, will become more saline [2]. Therefore, it is of great interest to study plant's physiological and metabolite responses to harsh environments where drought and salt stress are occurring simultaneously. However, only a few studies under this context have been performed [105–108]. Among them, only one study addressed maize metabolite responses induced by a combination of drought and salt stress [107]. Indeed, under its natural habitat of irrigated and dry land agricultural lands, maize is exposed to the combined stresses of water deficiency and soil salinity [107]. ^{1}H NMR-based metabolomics analysis of maize leaves revealed that metabolite responses of drought and salt stress differed from those caused by drought and salt stress applied individually. Additionally, subsequent multivariate statistical analysis allowed identifying those metabolites that specifically responded to the combined stress, namely two TCA cycle intermediates (citrate and fumarate) and four amino acids (the branched chain amino acids—valine, leucine and isoleucine, and the aromatic amino acid—phenylalanine) [107].

4.3. Metabolite responses to combined salt and heat stress

Up to date, studies on the combined effects of salt and heat stress in plants have revealed both positive and negative interactions on plant growth, yield and physiological traits (**Figure 2**). In wheat, the combination of salt and heat stress enhanced the transpiration rate, which in turn, was already induced by heat stress itself. On the other hand, this stress combination also promoted a higher uptake of Na^+ ions by the plant [109, 110].

The effects of the combination of salt and heat stress were evaluated in tomato plants (*Solanum lycopersicum* cv. Optima) [111]. This stress combination was observed to induce a specific response by the plants through the accumulation in the levels of glycine betaine and trehalose, both well-known for their osmoprotectant roles. The accumulation of glycine betaine and trehalose was associated to the maintenance of a lower Na^+:K^+ ratio, thereby leading to a better performance of the cell water status and photosynthesis when compared to the salt stress alone [111].

To the best of our knowledge, metabolomics studies aiming at dissecting metabolite responses induced by salt and heat stress are scarce, highlighting the need for further research in this area.

5. Concluding remarks

Climate change disturbs a number of variables that determine how much plants can grow and develop. Extreme temperatures, elevated CO_2 together with a decrease in water availability and changes to soil conditions will essentially make it more challenging for plants to thrive. Overall, climate change is expected to decline the growth and development of plants, particularly with reference to agricultural systems. Declining plant growth also dramatically changes the habitats that are necessary for many species to survive. Undoubtedly, under the current threat of climate change, it is urgent to address the molecular and biochemical mechanisms that underlie plant responses to several abiotic stresses and combinations thereof. However, a complete understanding of plant responses to climate change is best obtained if data is integrated at several levels, including morpho-physiological and developmental studies as well as molecular studies that comprise the so-called *omics* technologies. Up to now, metabolomics studies have already provided a promising basis for facilitating our understanding of the plant's flexibility to reconfigure central metabolic pathways (i.e., carbon, nitrogen and energy metabolism) as well as the degree by which plants tolerate and/or are susceptible to a climate change scenario. Nevertheless, more research efforts are crucial for a more comprehensive analysis of the impact of combined stresses in plants. Researchers must regard simultaneous multiple climate change factors, which sum will play a key negative influence on global agriculture, as a new state of stress in which the exposed plant might require differential responses from those induced by a stress alone. Further research in this area is therefore critical.

Acknowledgements

C. António gratefully acknowledges support from Fundação para a Ciência e a Tecnologia (FCT) through the FCT Investigator Program (IF/00376/2012/CP0165/CT0003) and from the ITQB NOVA research unit Green-IT "Bioresources for sustainability" (UID/Multi/04551/2013). T.F. Jorge acknowledges FCT for the PhD grant (PD/BD/113475/2015) from the ITQB NOVA International PhD program "Plants for Life" (PD/00035/2013).

Author details

Tiago F. Jorge and Carla António*

*Address all correspondence to: antonio@itqb.unl.pt

Plant Metabolomics Laboratory, Instituto de Tecnologia Química e Biológica António Xavier, Universidade Nova de Lisboa (ITQB NOVA), Oeiras, Portugal

References

[1] VijayaVenkataRamana S, Iniyanb S, Goic R. A review of climate change, mitigation and adaptation. Renewable & Sustainable Energy Reviews. 2012;**16**:878-897. DOI: 10.1016/j.rser.2011.09.009

[2] Core Writing Team IPCC. Climate Change 2014: Synthesis Report. Contribution of Working Groups I, II and III to the Fifth Assessment Report of the Intergovernmental Panel on Climate Change. Geneva: IPCC; 2014. 151 p

[3] Gray SB, Brady SM. Plant developmental responses to climate change. Developmental Biology. 2016;**419**:64-77. DOI: 10.1016/j.ydbio.2016.07.023

[4] Smith M. An ecological perspective on extreme climatic events: A synthetic definition and framework to guide future research. Journal of Ecology. 2011;**99**:656-663. DOI: 10.1111/j.1365-2745.2011.01798.x

[5] Becklin KM, Anderson JT, Gerhart LM, Wadgymar SM, Wessinger CA, Ward JK. Examining plant physiological responses to climate change through an evolutionary lens. Plant Physiology. 2016;**172**:635-649. DOI: 10.1104/pp.16.00793

[6] Felton AJ, Smith MD. Integrating plant ecological responses to climate extremes from individual to ecosystem levels. Philosophical Transactions of the Royal Society B. 2017;**372**:20160142. DOI: 10.1098/rstb.2016.0142

[7] Anderegg WRL, Kane JM, Anderegg LDL. Consequences of widespread tree mortality triggered by drought and temperature stress. Nature Climate Change. 2013;**3**:30-36. DOI: 10.1038/nclimate1635

[8] Bellard C, Bertelsmeier C, Leadley P, Thuiller W, Courchamp F. Impacts of climate change on the future of biodiversity. Ecology Letters. 2012;**15**:365-377. DOI: 10.1111/j.1461-0248.2011.01736.x

[9] Corlett RT, Westcott DA. Will plant movements keep up with climate change? Trends in Ecology & Evolution. 2013;**28**(8). DOI: 10.1016/j.tree.2013.04.003

[10] Franks SJ, Weber JJ, Aitken SN. Evolutionary and plastic responses to climate change in terrestrial plant populations. Evolutionary Applications. 2014;**7**:123-139. DOI: 10.1111/eva.12112

[11] Sulmon C, Baaren JV, Cabello-Hurtado F, Gouesbet G, Hennion F, Mony C, et al. Abiotic stressors and stress responses: What commonalities appear between species across biological organization levels? Environmental Pollution. 2015;**202**:66-77. DOI: 10.1016/j.envpol.2015.03.013

[12] Pacifici M, Foden WB, Visconti P, Watson JEM, Butchart SHM, Kovacs KM, et al. Assessing species vulnerability to climate change. Nature Climate Change. 2015;**5**:215-224. DOI: 10.1038/nclimate2448

[13] Palmer G, Platts PJ, Brereton T, Chapman JW, Dytham C, Fox R, et al. Climate change, climatic variation and extreme biological responses. Philosophical Transactions of the Royal Society B. 2017;**372**:20160144. DOI: 10.1098/rstb.2016.0144

[14] Hirayama T, Shinozaki K. Research on plant abiotic stress responses in the post-genome era: Past, present and future. The Plant Journal. 2010;**61**:1041-1052. DOI: 10.1111/j.1365-313X.2010.04124.x

[15] Pereira A. Plant abiotic stress challenges from the changing environment. Frontiers in Plant Science. 2011;**7**:1123. DOI: 10.3389/fpls.2016.01123

[16] Mittler R. Abiotic stress, the field environment and stress combination. Trends in Plant Science. 2006;**11**:15-19. DOI: 10.1016/j.tplants.2005.11.002

[17] Suzuki N, Rivero RM, Shulaev V, Blumwald E, Mittler R. Abiotic and biotic stress combinations. The New Phytologist. 2014;**203**:32-43. DOI: 10.1111/nph.12797

[18] Fiehn O, Kopka J, Dörmann P, Trethewey RN, Willmitzer L. Metabolite profiling for plant functional genomics. Nature Biotechnology. 2000;**18**:1157-1161. DOI: 10.1038/81137

[19] Fiehn O. Combining genomics, metabolome analysis and biochemical modelling to understand metabolic networks. Comparative and Functional Genomics. 2001;**2**:155-168. DOI: 10.1002/cfg.82

[20] Fiehn O. Metabolomics - the link between genotypes and phenotypes. Plant Molecular Biology. 2002;**48**:155-171. DOI: 10.1023/A:1013713905833

[21] Weckwerth W. Metabolomics in systems biology. Annual Review of Plant Biology. 2003;**54**:669-689. DOI: 10.1146/annurev.arplant.54.031902.135014

[22] Bino RJ, Hall RD, Fiehn O, Kopka J, Saito K, Draper J, et al. Potential of metabolomics as a functional genomics tool. Trends in Plant Science. 2004;**9**:418-425. DOI: 10.1016/j.tplants.2004.07.004

[23] Saito K, Matsuda F. Review metabolomics for functional genomics, systems biology, and biotechnology. Annual Review of Plant Biology. 2010;**61**:463-489. DOI: 10.1146/annurev.arplant.043008.092035

[24] Jorge TF, Rodrigues JA, Caldana C, Schmidt R, van Dongen JT, Thomas-Oates J, et al. Mass spectrometry-based plant metabolomics: Metabolite responses to abiotic stress. Mass Spectrometry Reviews. 2016;**35**:620-649. DOI: 10.1002/mas.21449

[25] Kopka J, Fernie A, Weckwerth W, Gibon Y, Stitt M. Metabolite profiling in plant biology: Platforms and destinations. Genome Biology. 2004;**5**:109.1-109.9. DOI: 10.1186/gb-2004-5-6-109

[26] Kopka J. Current challenges and developments in GC-MS based metabolite profiling technology. Journal of Biotechnology. 2006;**124**:312-322. DOI: 10.1016/j.jbiotec.2005.12.012

[27] Kopka J. Gas chromatography mass spectrometry. In: Saito K, Dixon RA, Willmitzer L, editors. Biotechnology in Agriculture and Forestry: Plant Metabolomics. Vol. 57. Berlin Heidelberg: Springer-Verlag; 2006. pp. 3-20. DOI: 10.1007/3-540-29782-0_1

[28] Fernie A. Metabolome characterisation in plant system analysis. Functional Plant Biology. 2003;**30**:111-120. DOI: 10.1071/FP02163

[29] Kim HK, Choi YH, Verpoorte R. NMR-based metabolomic analysis of plants. Nature Protocols. 2010;**5**:536-549. DOI: 10.1038/nprot.2009.237

[30] Kim HK, Choi YH, Verpoorte R. NMR-based plant metabolomics: Where do we stand, where do we go? Trends in Biotechnology. 2011;**29**:267-275. DOI: 10.1016/j.tibtech.2011.02.001

[31] Obata T, Fernie AR. The use of metabolomics to dissect plant responses to abiotic stresses. Cellular and Molecular Life Sciences. 2012;**69**:3225-3243. DOI: 10.1007/s00018-012-1091-5

[32] Kim HK, Verpoorte R. Sample preparation for plant metabolomics. Phytochemical Analysis. 2010;**21**:4-13. DOI: 10.1002/pca.1188

[33] Allwood JW, De Vos RCH, Moing A, Deborde C, Erban A, Kopka J, et al. Plant metabolomics and its potential for systems biology research: Background concepts, technology, and methodology. In: Jameson D, Verma M, Westerhoff H, editors. Methods in Enzymology. Vol. 500. Amsterdam: Academic Press; 2011. pp. 299-336. DOI: 10.1016/B978-0-12-385118-5.00016-5

[34] Jorge TF, Mata AT, António C. Mass spectrometry as a quantitative tool in plant metabolomics. Philosophical Transactions of the Royal Society A. 2016;**374**:20150370. DOI: 10.1098/rsta.2015.0370

[35] Chaves MM, Pereira JS, Maroco J, Rodrigues ML, Ricardo CP, Osório ML, et al. How plants cope with water stress in the field? Photosynthesis and growth. Annals of Botany. 2002;**89**:907-916. DOI: 10.1093/aob/mcf105

[36] Chaves MM, Maroco JP, Pereira JS. Understanding plant responses to drought – From genes to the whole plant. Functional Plant Biology. 2003;**30**:239-264. DOI: 10.1071/FP02076

[37] Chaves MM, Oliveira MM. Mechanisms underlying plant resilience to water deficits: Prospects for water-saving agriculture. Journal of Experimental Botany. 2004;**55**:2365-2384. DOI: 10.1093/jxb/erh269

[38] Tardieu F, Reymond M, Hamard P, Granier C, Muller B. Spatial distributions of expansion rate, cell division rate and cell size in maize leaves: A synthesis of the effects of soil water status, evaporative demand and temperature. Journal of Experimental Botany. 2010;**51**:1505-1514. DOI: 10.1093/jexbot/51.350.1505

[39] Bray EA. Genes commonly regulated by water-deficit stress in *Arabidopsis thaliana*. Journal of Experimental Botany. 2004;**55**:2331-2341. DOI: 10.1093/jxb/erh270

[40] Xue GP, McIntyre CL, Glassop D, Shorter R. Use of expression analysis to dissect alterations in carbohydrate metabolism in wheat leaves during drought stress. Plant Molecular Biology. 2008;**67**:197-214. DOI: 10.1007/s11103-008-9311-y

[41] Slama I, Abdelly C, Bouchereau A, Flowers T, Savoure A. Diversity, distribution and roles of osmoprotective compounds accumulated in halophytes under abiotic stress. Annals of Botany. 2015;**115**:433-447. DOI: 10.1093/aob/mcu239

[42] Mata AT, Jorge TF, Pires MV, António C. Drought stress tolerance in plants: Insights from metabolomics. In: Hossain MA, Wani SH, Bhattachajee S, Burritt DJ, Phan Tran LS, editors. Molecular and Genetic Perspectives. Vol. 2. Switzerland: Springer Publishing; 2016. pp. 187-216. DOI: 10.1007/978-3-319-32423-4_7

[43] Bartoli CG, Gomez F, Martinez DE, Guiamet JJ. Mitochondria are the main target for oxidative damage in leaves of wheat (*Triticum aestivum* L.). Journal of Experimental Botany. 2004;**55**:1663-1669. DOI: 10.1093/jxb/erh199

[44] Møller IM, Sweetlove LJ. ROS signaling – Specificity is required. Trends in Plant Science. 2010;**15**:370-374. DOI: 10.1016/j.tplants.2010.04.008

[45] Mittler R. Oxidative stress, antioxidants and stress tolerance. Trends in Plant Science. 2002;**7**:405-410. DOI: 10.1016/S1360-1385(02)02312-9

[46] Apel K, Hirt H. Reactive oxygen species: Metabolism, oxidative stress, and signal transduction. Annual Review of Plant Biology. 2004;**55**:373-399. DOI: 10.1146/annurev.arplant.55.031903.141701

[47] Baxter A, Mittler R, Suzuki N. ROS as key players in plant stress signaling. Journal of Experimental Botany. 2013;**65**:1229-1240. DOI: 10.1093/jxb/ert375

[48] Fukushima A, Kusano M, Redestig H, Arita M, Saito K. Integrated omics approaches in plant systems biology. Current Opinion in Chemical Biology. 2009;**13**:532-538. DOI: 10.1016/j.cbpa.2009.09.022

[49] Urano K, Kurihara Y, Seki M, Shinozaki K. 'Omics' analyses of regulatory networks in plant abiotic stress responses. Current Opinion in Plant Biology. 2010;**13**:132-138. DOI: 10.1016/j.pbi.2009.12.006

[50] Gupta B, Sengupta A, Saha J, Gupta K. Plant abiotic stress: 'Omics' approach. Journal of Plant Biochemistry & Physiology. 2013;**1**:1-2. DOI: 10.4172/2329-9029.1000e108

[51] Gechev T, Benina M, Obata T, Tohge T, Sujeeth N, Minkov I, et al. Molecular mechanisms of desiccation tolerance in the resurrection glacial relic Haberlea Rhodopensis. Cellular and Molecular Life Sciences. 2013;**70**:689-709. DOI: 10.1007/s00018-012-1155-6

[52] Yobi A, Wone BW, Xu W, Alexander DC, Guo L, Ryals JA, et al. Metabolomic profiling in Selaginella Lepidophylla at various hydration states provides new insights into the mechanistic basis of desiccation tolerance. Molecular Plant. 2013;**6**:369-385. DOI: 10.1093/mp/sss155

[53] Do PT, Degenkolbe T, Erban A, Heyer AG, Kopka J, Köhl KI, et al. Dissecting rice polyamine metabolism under controlled long-term drought stress. PLoS One. 2013;**8**:e60325. DOI: 10.1371/journal.pone.0060325

[54] Meyer E, Aspinwall MJ, Lowry DB, Palacio-Mejía JD, Logan TL, A Fay PA, et al. Integrating transcriptional, metabolomic, and physiological responses to drought stress and recovery in switchgrass (*Panicum virgatum* L.). BMC Genomics. 2014;**15**(1):**527**. DOI: 10.1186/1471-2164-15-527

[55] Chmielewska K, Rodziewicz P, Swarcewicz B, Sawikowska A, Krajewski P, Marczak Ł, et al. Analysis of drought-induced proteomic and metabolomic changes in barley (*Hordeum vulgare* L.) leaves and roots unravels some aspects of biochemical mechanisms involved in drought tolerance. Frontiers in Plant Science. 2016;**7**:1108. DOI: 10.3389/fpls.2016.01108

[56] Moschen S, Di Rienzo JA, Higgins J, Tohge T, Watanabe M, González S, et al. Integration of transcriptomic and metabolic data reveals hub transcription factors involved in drought stress response in sunflower (*Helianthus annuus* L.). Plant Molecular Biology. 2017;**94**:549-564. DOI: 10.1007/s11103-017-0625-5

[57] Goufo P, Moutinho-Pereira JM, Jorge TF, Correia CM, Oliveira MR, Rosa EAS, et al. Cowpea (*Vigna unguiculata* L. Walp.) metabolomics: Osmoprotection as a physiological strategy for drought stress resistance and improved yield. Frontiers in Plant Science. 2017;**8**:586. DOI: 10.3389/fpls.2017.00586

[58] Qadir M, Quillérou E, Nangia V, Murtaza G, Singh M, Thomas RJ, et al. Economics of salt-induced land degradation and restoration. Natural Resources Forum. 2014;**38**:282-295. DOI: 10.1111/1477-8947.12054

[59] Munns R, Tester M. Mechanisms of salinity tolerance. Annual Review of Plant Biology. 2008;**59**:651-681. DOI: 10.1146/annurev.arplant.59.032607.092911

[60] Chen TW, Kahlen K, Stutzel H. Disentangling the contributions of osmotic and ionic effects of salinity on stomatal mesophyll, biochemical and light limitations to photosynthesis. Plant, Cell & Environment. 2015;**38**:1528-1542. DOI: 10.1111/pce.12504

[61] Hasegawa PM, Bressan RA, Zhu JK, Bohnert HJ. Plant cellular and molecular responses to high salinity. Annual Review of Plant Physiology and Plant Molecular Biology. 2000; **51**:463-499. DOI: 10.1146/annurev.arplant.51.1.463

[62] Sanchez DH, Siahpoosh MR, Roessner U, Udvardi M, Kopka J. Plant metabolomics reveals conserved and divergent metabolic responses to salinity. Physiologia Plantarum. 2008;**132**:209-219. DOI: 10.1111/j.1399-3054.2007.00993.x

[63] Shulaev V, Cortes D, Miller G, Mittler R. Metabolomics for plant stress response. Physiologia Plantarum. 2008;**132**:199-208. DOI: 10.1111/j.1399-3054.2007.01025.x

[64] Sanchez DH, Pieckenstain FL, Escaray F, Erban A, Kraemer U, Udvardi MK, et al. Comparative ionomics and metabolomics in extremophile and glycophytic lotus species under salt stress challenge the metabolic pre-adaptation hypothesis. Plant, Cell & Environment. 2011;**34**:605-617. DOI: 10.1111/j.1365-3040.2010.02266.x

[65] Gong Q, Li P, Ma S, Indu SR, Bohnert HJ. Salinity stress adaptation competence in the extremophile Thellungiella Halophila in comparison with its relative Arabidopsis Thaliana. The Plant Journal. 2005;**44**:826-839. DOI: 10.1111/j.1365-313X.2005.02587.x

[66] Widodo, Patterson JH, Newbigin E, Tester M, Bacic A, Roessner U. Metabolic responses to salt stress of barley (Hordeum Vulgare L.) cultivars, Sahara and clipper, which differ in salinity tolerance. Journal of Experimental Botany. 2009;**60**:4089-4103. DOI: 10.1093/jxb/erp243

[67] Wu D, Cai S, Chen M, Ye L, Chen Z, Zhang H, et al. Tissue metabolic responses to salt stress in wild and cultivated barley. PLoS One. 2013;**8**:e55431. DOI: 10.1371/journal.pone.0055431

[68] Zuther E, Koehl K, Kopka J. Comparative metabolome analysis of the salt response in breeding cultivars of Rice. In: Jenks MA, Hasegawa PM, Jain SM, editors. Advances in Molecular Breeding toward Drought and Salt Tolerance Crops. Berlin Heidelberg: Springer-Verlag; 2007. pp. 285-315. DOI: 10.1007/978-1-4020-5578-2_12

[69] Dias AD, Hill CB, Jayasinghe NS, Atieno J, Sutton T, Roessner U. Quantitative profiling of polar primary metabolites of two chickpea cultivars with contrasting responses to salinity. Journal of Chromatography B. 2015:**100**:1-13. DOI: 10.1016/j.jchromb.2015.07.002

[70] Richter JA, Erban A, Kopka J, Zörb C. Metabolic contribution to salt stress in two maize hybrids with contrasting resistance. Plant Science. 2015;**233**:107-115. DOI: 10.1016/j.plantsci.2015.01.006

[71] Pawlowski K, Demchenko KN. The diversity of actinorhizal symbiosis. Protoplasma. 2012;**249**:967-979. DOI: 10.1007/s00709-012-0388-4

[72] Zhong C, Mansour S, Nambiar-Veetil M, Boguz D, Franche C. Casuarina Glauca: A model tree for basic research in actinorhizal symbiosis. Journal of Biosciences. 2013;**38**:815-823. DOI: 10.1007/s12038-013-9370-3

[73] Jorge TF, Duro N, da Costa M, Florian A, Ramalho JC, Ribeiro-Barros AI, et al. GC-TOF-MS analysis reveals salt stress-responsive primary metabolites in Casuarina Glauca tissues. Metabolomics. 2017;**13**:95. DOI: 10.1007/s11306-017-1234-7

[74] Duro N, Batista-Santos P, da Costa M, Maia R, Castro IV, Ramos M, et al. The impact of salinity on the symbiosis between Casuarina Glauca Sieb. Ex Spreng. And N2-fixing Frankia bacteria based on the analysis of nitrogen and carbon metabolism. Plant and Soil. 2016;**398**:327-337. DOI: 10.1007/s11104-015-2666-3

[75] Wahid A, Gelani S, Ashraf M, Foolad MR. Heat tolerance in plants: An overview. Environmental and Experimental Botany. 2007;**61**:199-223. DOI: 10.1016/j.envexpbot.2007.05.011

[76] Mittler R, Finka A, Goloubinoff P. How do plants feel the heat? Trends in Biochemical Sciences. 2012;**37**:118-125. DOI: 10.1016/j.tibs.2011.11.007

[77] Vierling E. The roles of heat shock proteins in plants. Annual Review of Plant Physiology and Plant Molecular Biology. 1991;**42**:579-620. DOI: 10.1146/annurev.pp.42.060191.003051

[78] Larkindale J, Vierling E. Core genome responses involved in acclimation to high temperature. Plant Physiology. 2008;**146**:748-761. DOI: 10.1104/pp.107.112060

[79] Kotak S, Larkindale J, Lee U, von Koskull-Döring P, Vierling E, Scharf KD. Complexity of the heat stress response in plants. Current Opinion in Plant Biology. 2007;**10**:310-316. DOI: 10.1016/j.pbi.2007.04.011

[80] Iba K. Acclimative response to temperature stress in higher plants: Approaches of gene engineering for temperature tolerance. Annual Review of Plant Biology. 2002;**53**:225-245. DOI: 10.1146/annurev.arplant.53.100201.160729

[81] Camejo D, Rodríguez P, Morales MA, Dell'amico JM, Torrecillas A, Alarcón JJ. High temperature effects on photosynthetic activity of two tomato cultivars with different heat susceptibility. Journal of Plant Physiology. 2005;**162**:281-289. DOI: 10.1016/j.jplph.2004.07.014

[82] Ahn YJ, Zimmerman JL. Introduction of the carrot HSP17.7 into potato (Solanum Tuberosum L.) enhances cellular membrane stability and tuberization in vitro. Plant, Cell & Environment. 2006;**29**:95-104. DOI: 10.1111/j.1365-3040.2005.01403.x

[83] Momcilovic I, Ristic Z. Expression of chloroplast protein synthesis elongation factor, EF-Tu, in two lines of maize with contrasting tolerance to heat stress during early stages of plant development. Journal of Plant Physiology. 2007;**164**:90-99. DOI: 10.1016/j.jplph.2006.01.010

[84] Bita CE, Gerats T. Plant tolerance to high temperature in a changing environment: Scientific fundamentals and production of heat stress-tolerant crops. Frontiers in Plant Science. 2013;**4**:273. DOI: 10.3389/fpls.2013.00273

[85] Hasanuzzaman M, Nahar K, Alam MM, Roychowdhury R, Fujita M. Physiological, biochemical, and molecular mechanisms of heat stress tolerance in plants. International Journal of Molecular Sciences. 2013;**14**:9643-9684. DOI: 10.3390/ijms14059643

[86] Wahid A, Close TJ. Expression of dehydrins under heat stress and their relationship with water relations of sugarcane leaves. Biologia Plantarum. 2007;**51**:104-109. DOI: 10.1007/s10535-007-0021-0

[87] Sato S, Kamiyama M, Iwata T, Makita N, Furukawa H, Ikeda H. Moderate increase of mean daily temperature adversely affects fruit set of Lycopersicon Esculentum by disrupting specific physiological processes in male reproductive development. Annals of Botany. 2006;**97**:731-738. DOI: 10.1093/aob/mcl037

[88] Du H, Wang Z, Yu W, Liu Y, Huang B. Differential metabolic responses of perennial grass Cynodon transvaalensis × Cynodon dactylon (C4) and Poa Pratensis (C3) to heat stress. Physiologia Plantarum. 2011;**141**:251-264. DOI: 10.1111/j.1399-3054.2010.01432.x

[89] Li Z, Yu J, Peng Y, Huang B. Metabolic pathways regulated by γ-aminobutyric acid (GABA) contributing to heat tolerance in creeping bentgrass (Agrostis Stolonifera). Scientific Reports. 2017;**6**:30338. DOI: 10.1038/srep30338 (2016)

[90] Pandey P, Ramegowda V, Senthil-Kumar M. Shared and unique responses of plants to multiple individual stresses and stress combinations: Physiological and molecular mechanisms. Frontiers in Plant Science. 2015;**6**:723. DOI: 10.3389/fpls.2015.00723

[91] Rizhsky L, Liang H, Mittler R. The combined effect of drought stress and heat shock on gene expression in tobacco. Plant Physiology. 2002;**130**:1143-1151. DOI: 10.1104/pp.006858

[92] Rizhsky L, Liang H, Shuman J, Shulaev V, Davletova S, Mittler R. When defense pathways collide. The response of Arabidopsis to a combination of drought and heat stress. Plant Physiology. 2004;**134**:1683-1696. DOI: 10.1104/pp.103.033431

[93] Zandalinas SI, Mittler R, Balfagón D, Arbona V, Gómez-Cadenas A. Plant adaptations to the combination of drought and high temperatures. Physiologia Plantarum. DOI: 10.1111/ppl.12540

[94] Koussevitzky S, Suzuki N, Huntington S, Armijo L, Sha W, Cortes D, et al. Ascorbate peroxidase 1 plays a key role in the response of Arabidopsis Thaliana to stress combination. The Journal of Biological Chemistry. 2008;**283**:34197-34203. DOI: 10.1074/jbc.M806337200

[95] Atkinson NJ, Lilley CJ, Urwin PE. Identification of genes involved in the response of Arabidopsis to simultaneous biotic and abiotic stresses. Plant Physiology. 2013;**162**:2028-2041. DOI: 10.1104/pp.113.222372

[96] Iyer NJ, Tang Y, Mahalingam R. Physiological, biochemical and molecular responses to a combination of drought and ozone in *Medicago truncatula*. Plant, Cell & Environment. 2013;**36**:706-720. DOI: 10.1111/pce.12008

[97] Prasch CM, Sonnewald U. Simultaneous application of heat, drought, and virus to Arabidopsis plants reveals significant shifts in signalling networks. Plant Physiology. 2013;**162**:1849-1866. DOI: 10.1104/pp.113.221044

[98] Rasmussen S, Barah P, Suarez-Rodriguez MC, Bressendorff S, Friis P, Costantino P, et al. Transcriptome responses to combinations of stresses in Arabidopsis. Plant Physiology. 2013;**161**:1783-1794. DOI: 10.1104/pp.112.210773

[99] Mittler R, Blumwald E. Genetic engineering for modern agriculture: Challenges and perspectives. Annual Review of Plant Biology. 2010;**61**:443-462. DOI: 10.1146/annurev-arplant-042809-112116

[100] Mittler R, Merquiol E, Hallak-Herr E, Rachmilevitch S, Kaplan A, Cohen M. Living under a "dormant" canopy: A molecular acclimation mechanism of the desert plant Retama raetam. The Plant Journal. 2001;**25**:407-416. DOI: 10.1046/j.1365-313x.2001.00975.x

[101] Zhang H, Sonnewald U. Differences and commonalities of plant responses to single and combined stresses. The Plant Journal. 2017;**90**:839-855. DOI: 10.1111/tpj.13557

[102] Obata T, Witt S, Lisec J, Palacios-Rojas N, Florez-Sarasa I, Araus JL, et al. Metabolite profiles of maize leaves in drought, heat and combined stress field trials reveal the relationship between metabolism and grain yield. Plant Physiology. 2015;**169**:2665-2683. DOI: 10.1104/pp.15.01164

[103] Jin R, Wang Y, Liu R, Gou J, Chan Z. Physiological and metabolic changes of purslane (*Portulaca oleracea* L.) in response to drought, heat, and combined stresses. Frontiers in Plant Science. 2016;**6**:1123. DOI: 10.3389/fpls.2015.01123

[104] Das A, Rushton PJ, Rohila JS. Metabolomic profiling of soybeans (Glycine max L.) reveals the importance of sugar and nitrogen metabolism under drought and heat stress. Plants. 2017;**6**:21. DOI: 10.3390/plants6020021

[105] Ahmed IM, Dai H, Zheng W, Cao F, Zhang G, Sun D, et al. Genotypic differences in physiological characteristics in the tolerance to drought and salinity combined stress between Tibetan wild and cultivated barley. Plant Physiology and Biochemistry. 2012;**63**:49-60. DOI: 10.1016/j.plaphy.2012.11.004

[106] Ahmed IM, Nadira UA, Bibi N, Cao F, He X, Zhang G, et al. Secondary metabolism and antioxidants are involved in the tolerance to drought and salinity, separately and combined, in Tibetan wild barley. Environmental and Experimental Botany. 2015;**111**:1-12

[107] Sun CX, Li MQ, Gao XX, Liu LN, XF W, Zhou JH. Metabolic response of maize plants to multi-factorial abiotic stresses. Plant Biology. 2016;**18**:120-129. DOI: 10.1111/plb.12305

[108] Nxele X, Klein A, Ndimba BK. Drought and salinity stress alters ROS accumulation, water retention, and osmolyte content in sorghum plants. South African Journal of Botany. 2017;**108**:261-266. DOI: 10.1016/j.sajb.2016.11.003

[109] Keles Y, Oncel I. Response of antioxidative defence system to temperature and water stress combinations in wheat seedlings. Plant Science. 2002;**163**:783-790. DOI: 10.1016/S0168-9452(02)00213-3

[110] Wen X, Qiu N, Lu Q, Lu C. Enhanced thermotolerance of photosystem II in salt-adapted plants of the halophyte Artemisia anethifolia. Planta. 2005;**220**:486-497. DOI: 10.1007/s00425-004-1382-7

[111] Rivero RM, Mestre TC, Mittler R, Rubio F, Garcia-Sanchez F, Martinez V. The combined effect of salinity and heat reveals a specific physiological, biochemical and molecular responses in tomato plants. Plant, Cell & Environment. 2014;**37**:1059-1073. DOI: 10.1111/pce.12199

Chapter 7

Integrated Chemical Control of Abiotic Stress Tolerance Using Biostimulants

Yasuo Yamauchi

Additional information is available at the end of the chapter

http://dx.doi.org/10.5772/intechopen.74214

Abstract

Given the high sensitivity of plants to environmental stress, the extreme environmental conditions derived from global climate change are now leading to a risk of decreases in crop production. The use of biostimulants, which enhance stress tolerance in plants, in combination with more traditional countermeasures, such as fertilizer application and irrigation, has significant potential to overcome stress-derived impacts on crops. In this review, the reasons for the inherent sensitivity of plants to environmental stress and the effects of biostimulants on enhancing stress tolerance are introduced. The availability of methods of integrated chemical control for improving crop production in the context of environmental stress is also discussed.

Keywords: abiotic stress, biostimulant, chemical control

1. Introduction

Global climate change means that extreme environmental conditions are now being experienced more frequently. The Intergovernmental Panel on Climate Change [1] has suggested that global warming increases the incidence of various natural disasters, such as extreme temperatures, flood, and drought; agriculture is particularly susceptible to the influence of such events, because plants are organisms that show great sensitivity to changes in their environment.

As sessile organisms, plants are constantly exposed to widely varying and unfavorable environmental conditions, such as drought and extreme temperatures, which are major limiting factors in crop production [2]. Plants therefore have an inherently complicated response mechanism against environmental stresses, including developmental, physiological, and biochemical changes that are regulated by abiotic-related gene expression. In this response process, environmental physical stimuli are perceived and transduced to biochemical processes, resulting in the induction of a series of abiotic stress-related gene expressions. The involvement of chemicals such as phytohormones, abscisic acid (ABA), salicylic acid (SA), jasmonic acid (JA), and ethylene has been shown to be important in the stress signaling process [3]. In addition, recent research suggests that a central role in the various causes of environmental stress is played by oxidized chemicals, which are produced in response to oxidative stress, an unavoidable stress for plants.

Stress-related disturbance of the metabolic balance in oxidative organelles often results in the enhanced production of reactive oxygen species (ROS) [4]. The sensitivity of plants to environmental stress partly arises because the cause of the damage derived from almost all abiotic stressors is related to photosynthesis. In terms of plant energy metabolism, photosynthesis is the process that is most sensitive in the presence of abiotic stress, because any imbalance between energy production in photochemical reactions and energy consumption in the Calvin-Benson cycle is often a result. As shown in **Figure 1**, the rate of photochemical reactions is almost dependent on a linear function with light intensity, because the photochemical reactions are mirrored

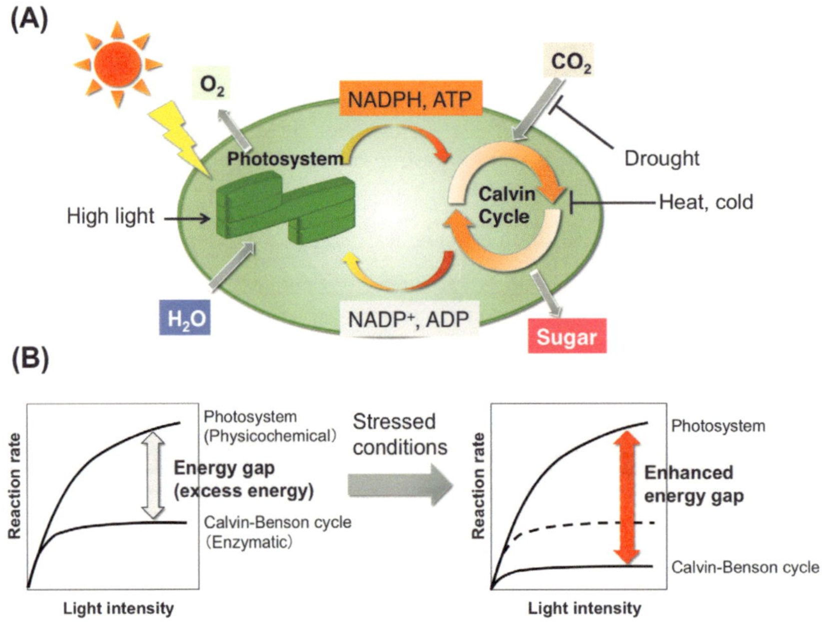

Figure 1. Chloroplasts comprise the most sensitive site in plants in responding to various environmental stresses. (A) Photosynthesis comprises two distinct processes: the photochemical reaction mediated by the photosystem, and CO_2 assimilation mediated by the Calvin-Benson cycle. Under environmental stresses such as high light levels, drought and temperature stresses, the NADPH and ATP supplied by photosystem and their consumption in the Calvin-Benson cycle become imbalanced [4]. (B) The energy gap between the photosystem and Calvin-Benson cycle is normally eliminated by thermal dissipation, but the energy imbalance occurred under environmental stresses enlarges the energy gap, often exceeding the dissipation capacity.

by physicochemical reactions. On the other hand, the Calvin-Benson cycle is a complex process comprising various enzymes; its rate is therefore restricted by enzymatic properties, such as the maximal velocity (V_{max}) value of each enzyme and the rate-limiting steps, and eventually reaches a plateau. Under balanced conditions such as low and moderate light intensity conditions, the quantity of NADPH and ATP supplied via the photosystem is almost equal to the $NADP^+$ and ADP returned from the Calvin-Benson cycle; this is not, however, the case under conditions of high light intensity, such as sunny weather. High light levels enhance photochemical reactions in the photosystem; in contrast, the Calvin-Benson cycle is inhibited by CO_2 deficiency under drought stress conditions, and its enzyme activity reduces under heat or cold conditions. When facing these stresses, the NADPH and ATP supplied by photosystem and their consumption in the Calvin-Benson cycle become imbalanced. This "energy gap," that is, the difference between energy supply and consumption, is usually eliminated by thermal energy dissipation. However, CO_2 deficiency due to stomatal closure under conditions of drought or high salinity, as well as enzyme inactivation during heat or cold stress, causes the rate of the Calvin-Benson cycle to lower, thereby increasing the energy gap. When this gap exceeds the capacity required for thermal energy to dissipate, the excess energy causes the production of ROS, potentially damaging many bioprocesses.

Consequently, disturbance of the photochemical reaction leads to the production of ROS, an effect that is further enhanced by conditions limiting CO_2 fixation, such as drought, salinity, heat and cold stress, and a combination of these conditions with high light intensity [4, 5]. ROS are primarily toxic compounds that damage cellular components because of their high reactivity, resulting in a decrease in plant production. Under oxidative stress conditions, ROS attack polyunsaturated fatty acids (PUFAs) in the thylakoid membrane; PUFAs are easily oxidized by ROS, releasing various degraded products. Malondialdehyde, which is representative of these degraded products and is easily produced by the oxidation of PUFAs [6], chemically modifies proteins, especially in conditions of high light intensity and heat stress [7]. Decreases in photosynthetic activity are partly due to the modification of malondialdehyde by reaction center proteins in photosystem II [8]. On the other hand, ROS [9], ROS-related chemicals such as carotenoid oxidation products [10], and lipophilic reactive electrophilic species [11] are recognized as important signal chemicals involved in the responses to environmental stress.

2. Potential chemicals involved in abiotic stress responses and their use as biostimulants

2.1. Reactive short-chain leaf volatiles as potential signaling chemicals

As described above, chloroplasts are the organelles that are most susceptible to damage under conditions of oxidative stress. Therefore, chloroplasts are also potential sensors of environmental stress, assimilating environmental changes, and transmitting information about the changes to other organelles using infochemicals. Recently, we have found evidence to support the premise that chloroplasts produce signal chemicals that induce gene expression and enhance stress tolerance.

Reactive short-chain leaf volatiles (RSLVs) are a group of C4–C9 straight chain carbonyls characterized by an α,β-unsaturated carbonyl bond (**Figure 2**). They are oxylipins and are derived from PUFAs in the thylakoid membrane. Biologically, plants treated with vaporized RSLVs show an enhanced expression of genes involved in responding to environmental stresses, such as high temperatures and oxidative stress [12]. As this response resembles the acquired thermotolerance inherent in plants as a response mechanism for surviving stress caused by elevated temperatures, plants treated with RSLVs show enhanced thermotolerance. As described later, the discovery of this bioactivity has opened the possibility of the chemical control of plants by volatiles to induce heat stress tolerance.

2.2. Improving crop production by enhancing environmental stress tolerance

In nature, crop yield is usually reduced by stress related to both biotic and abiotic causes; surprisingly, abiotic stress is the major inhibiting constraint, by up to 70% of potential production, in contrast to 10% for biotic stress (**Figure 3**, reconstituted from [13]). This indicates that crop production is on average only producing 20% of potential yield. Thus, if crop plants were liberated from abiotic stresses, by even only 10% of potential yield, then net crop production would increase by an average of 50%. Achieving this would be dependent on fertilizer-independent crop improvements, based on agriculturally beneficial biostimulants.

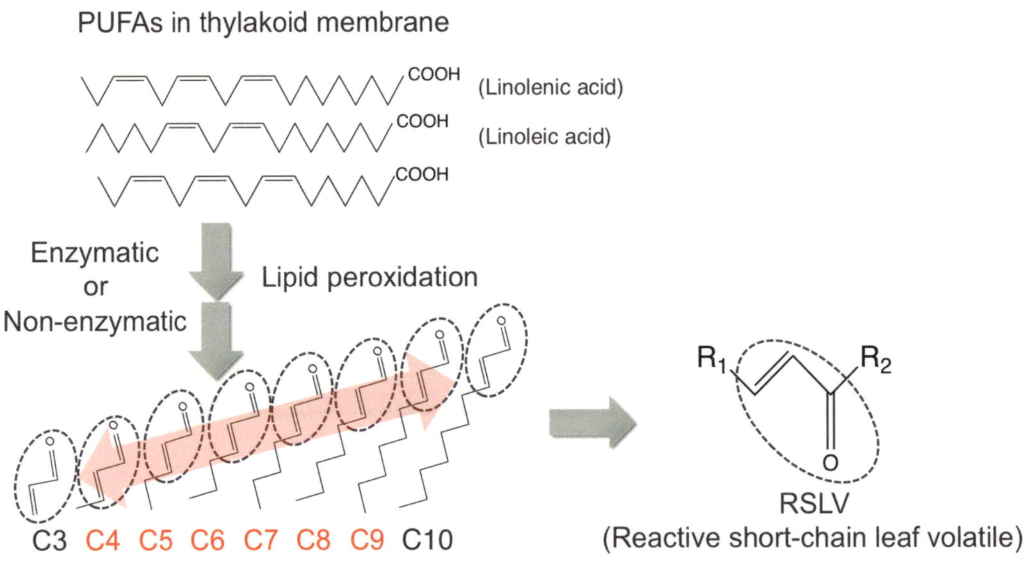

Figure 2. Reactive short-chain leaf volatiles (RSLVs) are signaling chemicals involved in the response to heat and oxidative stresses [12]. They are produced from oxidized polyunsaturated fatty acids, such as linolenic and linoleic acid, in thylakoid membranes through both enzymatic and nonenzymatic mechanisms. The essential chemical structure revealing signal activity is a straight chain carbonyl between C4 and C9, which has an α,β-unsaturated carbonyl bond (indicated by dotted circles). Of these, 2-hexenal is an RSLV produced enzymatically that is also known as a green leaf volatile.

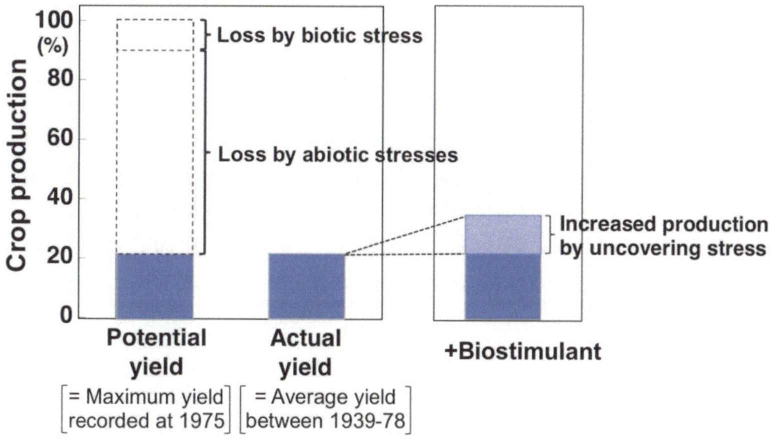

Figure 3. Concept of increase in crop production by using biostimulants. A comparison between the maximum yield recorded in 1975 (potential productivity) and average yield over a period of 50 years (1939–1978, actual productivity) shows that a large proportion of crop production is lost due to abiotic (up to 70%) and biotic (10%) stress (adapted from Table 1 in [13]). As shown in the right panel, if biostimulant treatment were to remove only 10% of the damage due to abiotic stress, net production would increase 1.5-fold when compared to no treatment being applied.

2.3. Use of biostimulants in enhancing tolerance to environmental stress

Crop yield has traditionally been improved by the application of fertilizers, pesticides, and irrigation to agricultural fields. Biostimulants are also products that have positive effects on yield by increasing stress tolerance and repairing damage already caused by unfavorable conditions [14, 15]. They can be either natural or synthetic in origin and usually consist of various organic and inorganic components. Naturally derived biostimulants include preparations based on free amino acids, seaweed and fruit extracts, effective microorganisms, humic substances, and chitosan [14, 15]. Synthetic biostimulants include plant growth regulators, phenolic compounds, inorganic salts, essential elements, and other substances with plant-stimulating properties. Hereafter, in this chapter, some major biostimulants, in particular chemical biostimulants with the potential to mitigate the effects of environmental stresses, are introduced.

2.4. Use of Pyrabactin as an ABA derivative for controlling water use

Under drought-stress conditions, plants often produce elevated levels of ABA to reduce transpiration by closing the guard cell aperture, resulting in a reduction in water loss. In order to control water use by plants, ABA derivatives have therefore been developed to activate the ABA receptors. Pyrabactin is representative of these synthetic ABA derivatives that mimic ABA; it activates the ABA receptors needed for improving drought tolerance [16]. Unlike natural ABA, Pyrabactin is not sensitive to light, is easy to synthesize, and relatively inexpensive, and its manufacture for agricultural use is therefore practical.

2.5. Acetic acid

The external application of acetate enhances drought tolerance in various plant species, such as *Arabidopsis*, maize, rapeseed, rice, and wheat [17]. This effect is related to a novel drought tolerance mechanism in plants involving the acetate-jasmonate signaling pathway, which is regulated epigenetically and conserved in plants. In *Arabidopsis*, exogenous acetic acid promotes JA synthesis and enriches histone H4 acetylation using ON/OFF switching, which is dependent on histone deacetylase HDA6, influencing the priming of the JA signaling pathway for plant drought tolerance. Thus, the external application of acetate to crops is potentially a useful, simple, and low-cost method of enhancing drought tolerance in various plant species.

2.6. Nonprotein amino acids and derivatives

The nonprotein amino acid β-aminobutyric acid (BABA), a potent inducer of resistance to infection by various pathogens [18], exerts its functions via priming of the SA-dependent defense mechanisms in Arabidopsis [19]. In other cases, BABA acts through potentiation of the ABA-dependent signaling pathways [20]. As both pathways can contribute to water stress tolerance, BABA is also able to protect Arabidopsis against abiotic stress, such as drought and high salinity [21], although BABA is a rare amino acid in plants [18]. This result suggests that BABA can be used as a biostimulant to protect plants from drought and salinity stress when it is based on ABA-dependent but not on SA-dependent defense mechanisms.

Glycine betaine is a major organic osmolyte that accumulates in various plant species in response to stresses such as drought and salinity [22]. It is an endogenous osmolyte produced by two enzymes: choline monooxygenase converts choline to betaine aldehyde, which is then catalyzed by betaine aldehyde dehydrogenase to form glycine betaine. As an osmolyte, glycine betaine is considered to have positive effects on the enzyme and membrane integrity in plants growing under stressful conditions; its role as a biostimulant has been subjected to field tests, and it is already being produced commercially. However, although many plant species show a significant increase in growth and final crop yield under conditions of environmental stress when treated with glycine betaine, others do not. Thus, the most useful and economic application of these compounds requires further investigations in order to determine the most effective concentrations and number of applications, as well as the most responsive growth stage(s) of the plant.

2.7. Controlling cold tolerance by modifying membrane fluidity

There is a close correlation between the chilling sensitivity of plants and the level of unsaturated fatty acids in the phosphatidylglycerol (PG), a phospholipid found in the thylakoid membranes of the chloroplasts [23]. When glycerol-3-phosphate acyltransferase, a key enzyme in determining the extent of unsaturated fatty acids in PG, is overexpressed, then increases in the relative levels of saturated and monounsaturated fatty acids in PG have been shown to increase the sensitivity of tobacco plants to low temperatures during the growth of young seedlings and maturation of reproductive organs [24]. As increases in the unsaturation of fatty acids result in decreases in biomembrane rigidification, then chemicals that enhance membrane rigidification can be used to promote tolerance against cold-induced stress. Furuya et al. [25] suggest that a treatment of dimethyl sulfoxide, which is a membrane rigidifier, enhanced the cold acclimation of *Arabidopsis* by activating the MEKK1-MKK2-MPK4 cascade. These results indicate that chemicals modifying lipid fluidity are a possible means of cold adaptation in plants.

2.8. Nitrophenolates

Nitrophenolates are biostimulants and are already being manufactured commercially in Japan under the name Atonik, a synthetic product composed of three phenolic compounds: sodium *p*-nitrophenolate (0.3%), sodium *o*-nitrophenolate (0.2%), and sodium 5-nitroguaiacolate (0.1%), together with water. Atonik has been used successfully for many years in the cultivation of most globally important crops. Its mode of action is still not understood but might be involved in hormone regulation, nutrient uptake, and nitrogen metabolism [26]. Atonik therefore stimulates plant growth and development and contributes to enhancing biomass accumulation, increasing water uptake, protecting against drought, and mitigating stress due to noble metals.

2.9. Use of RSLVs as biostimulants

As described in Section 2.1, RSLVs potentially act as signaling chemicals involved in heat and oxidative responses. A representative RSLV, 2-hexenal, is a green leaf volatile that induces gene expression in response to heat and oxidative stresses [12] and thus enhances thermotolerance in plants. Terada et al. suggest that this effect is partly explained by transpiration being sustained at higher temperatures [27]. The field use of 2-hexenal is being progressed commercially in Japan. 2-hexenal is a volatile; its vaporization from a tablet form by sublimation has enabled the effective concentrations for use in closed greenhouses to be determined. A preliminary examination showed that its application in greenhouses improved the production of crops such as tomato, strawberry, and cucumber in the summer (unpublished data), suggesting that its use as a biostimulant is effective in overcoming heat stress.

3. Perspective: toward an integrated chemical control against environmental stress

Historically, the use of pesticides, irrigation, and fertilizers, especially chemical fertilizers, has proven highly successful in increasing crop yields and thus in meeting the demands of increasing population levels. However, recent climate change is having an adverse impact on crop production, and therefore, more efficient methods of crop production need to be established. The use of genetically modified organisms (GMOs) is undoubtedly a solution to combat losses in plant production caused by global environmental changes. However, GMO is limited to major crops, and its use is also either strictly restricted or not even permitted legally in several countries. Therefore, chemical control of abiotic stress tolerance is required as an alternative solution for ensuring unrestricted agricultural production.

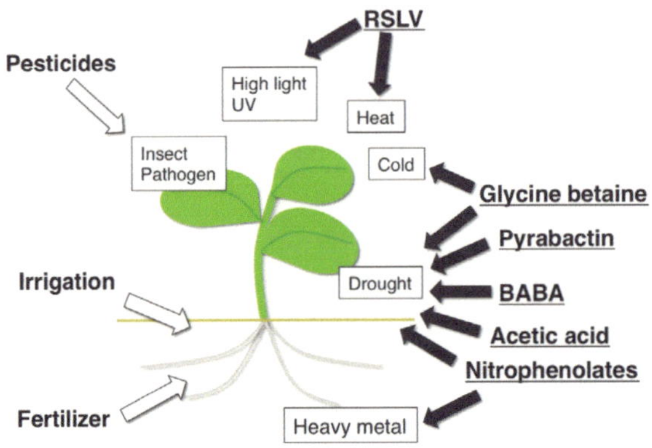

Figure 4. Integrated chemical control of abiotic stress tolerance using biostimulants. Traditional countermeasures, such as irrigation and fertilizers, contribute to improving the basal level of crop production. On the other hand, unusual losses in crop yield caused by biotic and abiotic stress can be mitigated by pesticides and biostimulants, respectively. In this figure, unusual adverse events and biostimulants are boxed and underlined, respectively. The stresses targeted by traditional countermeasures and biostimulants are indicated by white and black arrows, respectively.

As introduced in this chapter, the use of biostimulants has potential as a powerful countermeasure for improving crop production under conditions of environmental stress. Traditional methods for enhancing yield, such as fertilizer and irrigation support, enable a basal level of production to be maintained (**Figure 4**). However, when crops are subject to unusual abiotic and/or biotic stresses, the transient use of adequate biostimulant(s) helps to overcome these stresses, sustaining production to at least the basal level, and sometimes bringing about an increase in crop production, as explained in **Figure 3**. Some biostimulants are already commercially available, and their use will become increasingly popular. However, there is still a lack of technical information for each biostimulant, such as the application period, concentration, and target plant species; these points must be established if biostimulant application is to become a reliable technique. Moreover, the combined use of biostimulants and traditional pesticides must be examined in order to realize the integrated chemical control of abiotic/biotic stress tolerance. In addition to the chemical biostimulants that are the focus of this chapter, other types of biostimulants that are derived from natural materials, such as microorganisms and algae, are also useful in reducing damage caused by abiotic stress [14, 15]. While the mode of action in chemical biostimulants can be explained scientifically, this is not the case for natural biostimulants. Therefore, more details on scientific analyses of the mechanisms used by biostimulants are necessary to support their availability for widespread use in the field.

Acknowledgements

A part of unpublished data introduced in this chapter was generously provided by Phytochrome Inc. (Tokyo, Japan).

http://dx.doi.org/10.5772/intechopen.74214

Conflicts of interest

The authors declare no conflict of interest.

Abbreviations

ABA	abscisic acid
BABA	β-aminobutyric acid
GMO	genetically manipulated organism
JA	jasmonic acid
PG	phosphatidyl glycerol
PUFA	polyunsaturated fatty acid
ROS	reactive oxygen species
RSLV	reactive short-chain leaf volatile
SA	salicylic acid

Author details

Yasuo Yamauchi

Address all correspondence to: yamauchi@kobe-u.ac.jp

Graduate School of Agricultural Science, Kobe University, Kobe, Japan

References

[1] Porter JR, Xie L, Challinor AJ, Cochrane K, Howden SM, Iqbal MM, Lobell DB, Travasso MI, Chhetri N, Garrett K, Ingram J, Lipper L, McCarthy N, McGrath J, Smith D, Thornton P, Watson J, Ziska L. Food Security and food production systems. In: Field CB, Barros VR, Dokken DJ, Mach KJ, Mastrandrea MD, Bilir TE, Chatterjee M, Ebi KL, Estrada YO, Genova RC, Girma B, Kissel ES, Levy AN, MacCracken S, Mastrandrea PR, White LL, editors. Climate Change 2014: Impact, adaptation, and vulnerability. PartA: Global and sectoral aspects: Cambridge University Press; 2014. p. 485-533

[2] Fujita M, Fujita Y, Noutoshi Y, Takahashi F, Narusaka Y, Yamaguchi-Shinozaki K, Shinozaki K. Crosstalk between abiotic and biotic stress responses: a current view from the points

of convergence in the stress signaling networks. Current Opinion in Plant Biology. 2006;**9**:436-442. DOI: 10.1016/j.pbi.2006.05.014

[3] Scharf KD, Berberich T, Ebersberger I, Nover L. The plant heat stress transcription factor (Hsf) family: Structure, function and evolution. Biochimica et Biophysica Acta. 2012;**1819**:104-119. DOI: 10.1016/j.bbagrm.2011.10.002

[4] Asada K. The water-water cylce in chloroplasts: Scavenging of active oxygens and dissipation of excess photons. Annual Review of Plant Physiology and Plant Molecular Biology. 1999;**50**:601-639. DOI: 10.1146/annurev.arplant.50.1.601

[5] Mittler R. Abiotic stress, the field environment and stress combination. Trends in Plant Science. 2006;**11**:15-19. DOI: 10.1016/j.tplants.2005.11.002

[6] Esterbauer H, Schaur RJ, Zollner H. Chemistry and biochemistry of 4-hydroxynonenal, malonaldehyde and related aldehydes. Free Radical Biology and Medicine. 1991;**11**: 81-128. DOI: 10.1016/0891-5849(91)90192-6

[7] Yamauchi Y, Furutera A, Seki K, Toyoda Y, Tanaka K, Sugimoto Y. Malondialdehyde generated from peroxidized linolenic acid causes protein modification in heat-stressed plants. Plant Physiology and Biochemistry. 2008;**46**:786-793. DOI: 10.1016/j.plaphy.2008.04.018

[8] Yamauchi Y, Sugimoto Y. Effect of protein modification by malondialdehyde on the interaction between the oxygen-evolving complex 33 kDa protein and photosystem II core proteins. Planta. 2010;**231**:1077-1088. DOI: 10.1007/s00425-010-1112-2

[9] Scarpeci TE, Zanor MI, Carrillo N, Mueller-Roeber B, Valle EM. Generation of superoxide anion in chloroplasts of *Arabidopsis thaliana* during active photosynthesis: A focus on rapidly induced genes. Plant Molecular Biology. 2008;**66**:361-378. DOI: 10.1007/s11103-007-9274-4

[10] Ramel F, Birtic S, Ginies C, Soubigou-Taconnat L, Triantaphylidès C, Havaux M. Carotenoid oxidation products are stress signals that mediate gene responses to singlet oxygen in plants. Proceedings of the National Academy of Sciences of the United States of America. 2012;**109**:5535-5540. DOI: 10.1073/pnas.1115982109

[11] Farmer E, Davoine C. Reactive electrophile species. Current Opinion in Plant Biology. 2007;**10**:380-386. DOI: 10.1016/j.pbi.2007.04.019

[12] Yamauchi Y, Kunishima M, Mizutani M, Sugimoto Y. Reactive short-chain leaf volatiles act as powerful inducers of abiotic stress-related gene expression. Scientific Reports. 2015;**5**:8030. DOI: 10.1038/srep08030

[13] Boyer JS. Plant productivity and environment. Science. 1982;**218**:443-448. DOI: 10.1126/science.218.4571.443

[14] Calvo P, Nelson L, Kloepper JW. Agricultural uses of plant biostimulants. Plant and Soil. 2014;**383**:3-41. DOI: 10.1007/s11104-014-2131-8

[15] Van Oosten MJ, Pepe O, De Pascale S, Silletti S, Maggio A. The role of biostimulants and bioeffectors as alleviators of abiotic stress in crop plants. Chemical and Biological Technology in Agriculture. 2017;**4**:5. DOI: 10.1186/s40538-017-0089-5

[16] Park SY, Peterson FC, Mosquna A, Yao J, Volkman BF, Cutler SR. Agrochemical control of plant water use using engineered abscisic acid receptors. Nature. 2015;**520**:545-548. DOI: 10.1038/nature14123

[17] Kim JM, To TK, Matsui A, Tanoi K, Kobayashi IN, Matsuda F, Habu Y, Ogawa D, Sakamoto T, Matsunaga S, Bashir K, Rasheed S, Ando M, Takeda H, Kawaura K, Kusano M, Fukushima A, Endo TA, Kuromori T, Ishida J, Morosawa T, Tanaka M, Torii C, Takebayashi Y, Sakakibara H, Ogihara Y, Saito K, Shinozaki K, Devoto A, Seki M. Acetate-mediated novel survival strategy against drought in plants. Nature Plants. 2017;**3**:17097. DOI: 10.1038/nplants.2017.97

[18] Jakab G, Cottier V, Toquin V, Rigoli G, Zimmerli L, Metraux JP, Mauch-Mani B. β-Aminobutyric acid-induced resistance in plants. European Journal of Plant Pathology. 2001;**107**:29-37. DOI: 10.1023/A:1008730721037

[19] Zimmerli L, Jakab G, Metraux JP, Mauch-Mani B. Potentiation of pathogen-specific defense mechanisms in Arabidopsis by β-aminobutyric acid. Proceedings of the National Academy of Sciences USA. 2000;**97**:12920-12925. DOI: 10.1073/pnas.230416897

[20] Ton J, Mauch-Mani B. β-Amino-butyric acid-induced resistance against necrotrophic pathogens is based on ABA-dependent priming for callose. Plant Journal. 2004;**38**:119-130. DOI: 10.1111/j.1365-313X.2004.02028.x

[21] Jakab G, Ton J, Flors V, Zimmerli L, Métraux JP, Mauch-Mani B. Enhancing Arabidopsis salt and drought stress tolerance by chemical priming for its abscisic acid responses. Plant Physiology. 2005;**139**:267-274. DOI: 10.1104/pp.105.065698

[22] Ashraf M, Foolad MR. Roles of glycine betaine and proline in improving plant abiotic stress resistance. Environmental and Experimental Botany. 2007;**59**:206-216. DOI: 10.1016/j.envexpbot.2005.12.006

[23] Murata N. Molecular species composition of phosphatidylglycerol from chilling-sensitive and chilling-resistant plants. Plant and Cell Physiology. 1983;**24**:81-86. DOI: 10.1093/oxfordjournals.pcp.a076516

[24] Sakamoto A, Sulpice R, Hou CX, Kinoshita M, Higashi SI, Kanaseki T, Nonaka H, Moon BY, Murata N. Genetic modification of the fatty acid unsaturation of phosphatidylglycerol in chloroplasts alters the sensitivity of tobacco plants to cold stress. Plant Cell Environment. 2003;**27**:99-105. DOI: 10.1046/j.0016-8025.2003.01131.x

[25] Furuya T, Matsuoka D, Nanmori T. Membrane rigidification functions upstream of the MEKK1-MKK2-MPK4 cascade during cold acclimation in *Arabidopsis thaliana*. FEBS Letter. 2014;**588**:2025-2030. DOI: 10.1016/j.febslet.2014.04.032

[26] Przybysz A, Gawrońska H, Gajc-Wolska J. Biological mode of action of a nitrophenolates-based biostimulant: Case study. Frontiers in Plant Science. 2014;**5**:713. DOI: 10.3389/fpls.2014.00713

[27] Terada N, Sanada A, Gemma H, Koshio K. Effect of *trans*-2-hexenal vapor pretreatment on alleviation of heat stress of tomato seedlings (Micro Tom). Journal of ISSAAS. 2017;**23**:1-7

Chapter 8

Tolerance-Induction Techniques and Agronomical Practices to Mitigate Stress in Extensive Crops and Vegetables

Hipólito Hernández-Hernández,
Fabián Pérez-Labrada, Ema Laura García Enciso,
Paola Leija-Martínez, Mari Carmen López-Pérez,
Julia Medrano-Macías, Susana González-Morales,
Antonio Juárez Maldonado,
Luis Rubén García Dávila and
Adalberto Benavides Mendoza

Additional information is available at the end of the chapter

http://dx.doi.org/10.5772/intechopen.71771

Abstract

Environmental stress has regulated the function, morphology, and diversity of cells, organs, individuals and plant communities. The interaction of plants with the stress-inducing environments has produced in the plants a set of adaptive responses that can be studied in different description scopes: from organelles and subcellular structures to the level of plant communities. When it occurs for short time or low intensity, environmental stress can induce *hardening,* followed by induction of tolerance; on the other hand, when the plant's reaction is for a long time or responding to a significant stress intensity, the response of plants includes decreased growth, depletion of metabolic reserves and loss of productivity and yield, even reaching the death of plants. Current knowledge about these crop responses can be translated into agronomic practices aimed at mitigating the adverse effects of environmental stress. This chapter will present the mechanisms of response and adaptation of crop plants to the environmental factors that most commonly cause crop damage or yield loss: high and low temperature, salinity, water deficit and nutrient deficits. Agronomic practices aimed at modifying or balancing some of the environmental factors involved and the use of tolerance induction techniques are described.

Keywords: hardening, stress hardiness, biostimulation, abiotic stress, multiple stresses

1. Introduction

Climate change is a reality that we must address using technology, scientific knowledge, and economic and social policies that modify the relationship between human society and its environment. Climate change already represents a multifaceted challenge for the sustainable production of food, for health, and in general for the culture and current patterns of level and quality of life of humans [1]. In the particular case of food production through field crops (cereals, oilseeds, vegetables, etc.), the expected scenarios indicate the increasingly frequent occurrence of unfavorable climatic events to agricultural production. This non-benign scenario forces the agricultural production processes to be modified and adjusted to a new reality [2].

Different techniques of agricultural production, such as the use of protected spaces (greenhouses, shade cloth, tunnels, and mulching) [3], modern genetic modification techniques [4], the implementation of translational processes based on systems biology [5], and the large-scale implementation of vertical farms and plant factories [6] can provide some of the food needed for the growing human population. However, at this time getting the calories, minerals and fiber necessary for the feeding of humans and their domestic animals are still an enterprise carried out almost entirely on soils in the open field [3].

The shift to a system where 100% of the food for the population is produced on vertical farms and plant factories implies a profound change in the culture and food processes, such as reducing or eliminating meat consumption and food waste, among others [3]. Considering the above, it seems that crop production will still occur mostly using soils in open field production systems, so the expected greater magnitude of the stress associated with climate change does not seem to have a solution that depends entirely on the crop under protected conditions.

In any case, even with the expectation of having robotic systems, automation and abundant sources of energy, whether food production is carried out in the field, in a laboratory, or on a vertical farm or plant factory, in all the mentioned situations should be applied the concepts of sustainable production, care of natural resources, mitigation of environmental impact and pollution, since by definition any industrial process will have an impact on the environment [7]. On the other hand, even advanced industrial systems for food production such as vertical farms and plant factories depend on supplies such as water of a certain quality, high humidity in the air and an adequate range of temperatures for their cost-effective management, whose availability most likely will be dependent on processes associated with climate change and the modification of environmental services.

On the other hand, under climatic change, the adjustments in the traditional patterns of distribution of precipitation, temperature, and atmospheric humidity, among others, are inevitable. It is possible that a modification in the form of new climatic conditions will be reached at a global level, which will inevitably prevail over a period that may be extensive on a human scale, but fleet at the scale of the climatic processes of the terrestrial system. Such an adjustment surely involves winners and losers as to the circumstances of food production in some regions [2].

With the climate change process, adverse scenarios for agriculture and in general for the production of foods, fibers, and other plant-derived raw materials are seen more complicated by the greater intensity of stress-inducing events, their increasingly unpredictable nature, and the correlation with biotic-type stresses [8]. This manuscript describes a set of agronomic practices and tolerance induction techniques aimed at improving productivity, yield, and crop quality within an integrated soil-plant management strategy that takes into account both the highest intensity as well as the greater variety of environmental stresses.

2. Responses to multiple stresses

In plants for cultivation, stress always occurs in a combined form, that is to say, there is not a single type of stress in isolation [9, 10]. It is known that in the scope of the description of the transcriptome, proteome, and metabolome, the combination of different stresses gives rise to different response profiles to those observed in the case of individual stress [8, 11]. That is, from a molecular point of view, the combination of two or more stresses generates a unique expression profile, which has made difficult the progress in obtaining transgenic crops with tolerance to multiple stresses [12].

However, when moving from the molecular scale to the areas of cellular and physiological-morphological description, biochemical and process-modulated responses to multiple abiotic stresses present typical responses to different stresses and their combinations. Among these are the induction of antioxidants, signaling molecules, chelating agents, compatible solutes, or osmolytes, specific hormone balances, chaperone proteins, regulation of the amount of N and foliar chlorophyll, control of stomatal opening and photosynthetic activity, induction of energy dissipation activities such as photorespiration and xanthophyll cycle and changes in growth rate and root/shoot ratios, among others [13, 14].

The induction of responses to one or more stresses activates a series of defense responses that have been described in the molecular, cellular or physiological-morphological domain. When a seed, seedling or plant is subjected to a stress stimulus with a degree of intensity that does not cause extensive damage in individuals, or when the concentration of one or more of the metabolites involved in responses to stress (antioxidants, osmolytes, etc.) is increased by means of exogenous applications or genetic manipulation, a phenomenon of partial activation of plant defenses occurs known as *hardening*, which allows that a post-stress exposure to cause minor damage to plants. When hardening occurs by prior exposure to a different type of stress, it is referred to as *cross-resistance*. The hardening technique has been widely reported as a mechanism of induction of stress tolerance.

It is likely that the defense responses, which initially manifest at the level subcellular, and organelles, but with a later impact on the physiological-morphological domain of the whole organism, depend on changes in cellular redox balance, which are the result of oxidative damage and disorganization of the energy transfer and information network which obeys

Pre-sowing	Sowing or transplanting	Crop growth	Post-harvest	Stress factor in which tolerance is induced
Soil management: • Organic and mineral amendments • Cover crops • Low tillage • Crop rotation • Zeolites, nanofertilizers		*Soil management:* • Organic and mineral amendments • Low tillage • Nanofertilizers		High irradiance Water stress High temperature Salinity
Use of soil microorganisms: • Arbuscular mycorrhizal fungi and rhizobacteria				Water stress High temperature Salinity Mineral deficiency
Use of genetically improved plants: • Hybrid seeds (traditional breeding) • Transgenic crops • Genetic modification (non-transgenic)				High irradiance Water stress High and low temperature Salinity Mineral deficiency
Tolerance inductors and elicitors: • Organic compounds • Beneficial elements • Nanocompounds and nanofertilizers				High irradiance Water stress High and low temperature Salinity Mineral deficiency

Table 1. Use of management strategies in different stages of cultivation for abiotic stress mitigation in plants.

the structure of the membranes, their integral proteins and their interaction with the cytoskeleton [15]. In other organizational scopes, such as ecosystems, similar phenomena have been described where disruption in some system components (by example, a decline in biodiversity) has a negative impact on energy efficiency [16, 17].

The proper use of energy by a system is probably the primary process affected during a stressful situation. It is desirable and possible to moderate the damage caused by energy imbalance, not only at the molecular level but also in the description scope of cells, organisms, and ecosystems. At each level, appropriate measures would be applied, depending on the properties that can be manipulated in each scope. Each of the actions in the different fields would synergistically contribute to the mitigation of crop stress. These multiple approaches, which should ideally be comprehensive, contemplate different levels of description and response of the productive system and are expected to improve the ability to adapt and produce food under the climate change scenarios [18].

When stress is caused by multiple factors, it has been observed that the simultaneous application of several different mitigation measures results in a positive synergistic response of the plant [19]. Considering this, the application of agronomic practices aimed at the mitigation of the primary stresses for field crops can be carried out in two phases: the first one starting from the common component of stress due to excess PAR, the second considering the current knowledge about responses to stress in plants at the cellular and physiological level. The first phase refers to the management of the soil capacity to store water, to contribute CO_2 in a sustained way to the canopy of plants, and to maintain an abundant and biodiverse microbiome. The second phase refers to the potentially synergistic use of fertilizers, regulators, elicitors, and other chemicals to mitigate oxidative damage, in conjunction with tolerant varieties or landraces, irrigation systems, and tillage processes with less impact on the soil (**Table 1**). In an ideal situation, the practices mentioned for each phase should be applied simultaneously, although situations are also possible where only one part is applied, and positive results are obtained.

In this chapter, we present the measures that we propose to apply to the interaction domain of crop plants, soil, and atmosphere, that is, on the scale of an agricultural ecosystem. At this level (particularly in C3 species) the environmental factor irradiance seems to be a common confluence point for stress caused by multiple factors [20, 21]. As a consequence, mitigating the stress resulting from high levels of PAR in crop fields could reduce the impact of other stress-inducing environmental factors such as water deficit, salinity, and heat.

3. High irradiance stress

The management of the stress condition due to high irradiance, which is very common in C3 crops, depends on two main factors: the capacity of the edaphic system to contribute CO_2 and water in the time of maximum irradiance, as well as the efficiency of the photochemical and biochemical dissipation processes that produce thermal energy and ROS, in addition to the plant ability to reduce the impact of the products of dissipative processes on the biochemical and physiological processes that determine growth and reproduction. For the first factor, the key to management is the soil condition, especially the content of organic matter and the promotion of the microbiome of plants. Also, other measures can be applied such as the reduction of tillage, the use of high-efficiency irrigation systems and the use of hydrophilic polymers. For the second factor, the ability (intrinsic, improved, or genetically modified) to tolerate the stress of each species or variety is considered, as well as the use of various substances or mineral elements that function as tolerance inducers (such as Si, Se, and various nanomaterials of Fe, Zn, etc.), antioxidants, and substances or materials that modify foliar reflectance or the use of radiation (**Figure 1**).

3.1. Irradiance and CO_2 availability

Solar radiation is the primary source of energy for the photosynthetic process. With the current condition of atmospheric CO_2 concentration (400 μL L^{-1}), a significant part of the CO_2 used

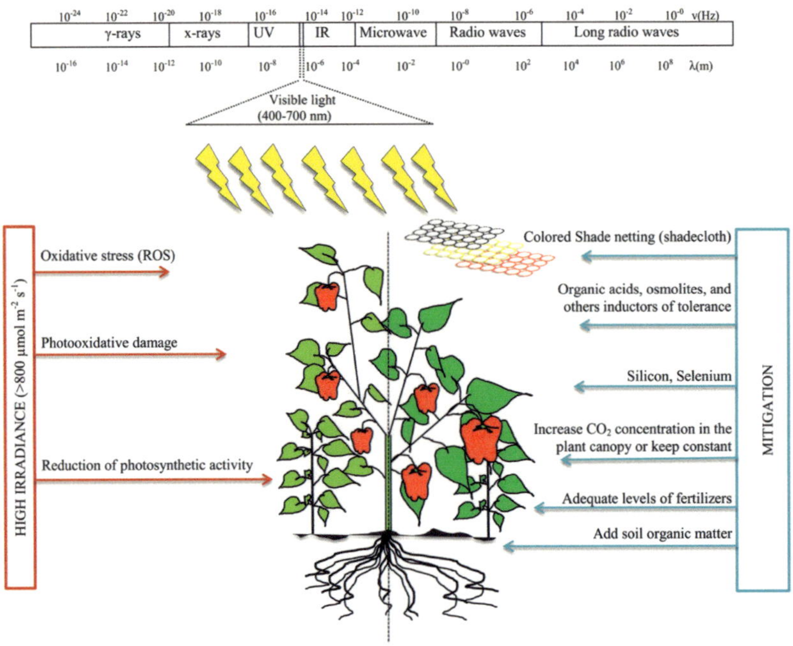

Figure 1. Oxidative components of high irradiance damage (left), and the factors for crop mitigation.

as a carbon source during photosynthesis comes from soil respiration, and in many cases, CO_2 deficiency is found in the canopy of plants during the hours when values of photosynthetic irradiance (PPFD) from 1800 to 2000 μmol m^{-2} s^{-1} are reached [22]. In this regard [23], mention that a PPFD of 600–800 μmol m^{-2} s^{-1} allow the adequate photosynthetic activity.

As PPFD values increase beyond 800 μmol m^{-2} s^{-1}, in combination with a low CO_2 content in the canopy, an increasing share of the energy captured by the leaves is not used for the photochemical reactions that produce ATP and $NADPH_2$ in the photosystems, but the excess energy is drifted toward the activation of O_2 by the triplet chlorophyll of the antennas or reaction centers to produce singlet oxygen ($^1O_2$), or is dissipated in processes of non-photochemical quenching that produce thermal radiation, fluorescence, or formation of free radicals. Singlet oxygen and other radicals such as superoxide (O_2^-) produced by photochemical systems can interact with membranes, proteins, and other biomolecules causing oxidative damage, which requires a high metabolic expenditure in the form of antioxidants for their control [23, 24]. On the other hand, the production of thermal energy increases the leaf temperature which promotes the loss of water by transpiration, increases the respiratory rate and decreases the volume of stored carbon available for growth [25]. This decline in leaf carbohydrates can have a profound impact on the nocturnal growth of the plant and the export of photosynthates to grains, fruits, and tubers.

The combination of high irradiance and low CO_2 concentration in the canopy results in the induction of photo-oxidative damage and higher foliar temperature, which, if not adequately controlled, cause a decrease in CO_2 assimilation capacity, a response associated with the increase in the stomatal resistance derived from the high transpiration rate, the decline in chlorophyll concentration, the reduction in RUBISCO activity and in the quantum yield of photosystems [23]. In conjunction with increased metabolic expenditure and higher respiratory rate, the result is less availability of photosynthates for growth and defense, which in turn decreases the ability to tolerate other abiotic or biotic stresses [26]. In turn, the drop in the number of photosynthates has an adverse impact on the capacity of the plant to assimilate N, since under sufficient conditions much of the N absorbed is used to be incorporated into amino acids and proteins, where RUBISCO one of the most abundant [27]. This adverse effect on N assimilation subsequently decreases the uptake and assimilation of other nutrients such as K, S, and P, causing nutritional imbalances in the plant [28].

As mentioned above, it is possible to alleviate stress induced by high PPDF if the irradiance is reduced or if the concentration of CO_2 in the canopy is increased and an adequate supply of water is ensured during the hours of greatest demand. In the photosynthetic process the CO_2 is used as the sink of the reducing potential produced by the photochemical reactions, so the way to channel more energy toward the photochemical reactions, decreasing the counterpart of non-photochemical quenching, is to increase the availability of CO_2 in the mesophyll of the leaf. Under conditions of high irradiance, the only way to achieve this result is by increasing the concentration of CO_2 in the canopy [14].

The reduction of PPDF is possible in some crops using neutral or colored shade cloths that decrease PPFD in different percentages [29], usually 15, 20, or 30%. However, the large-scale use of shade cloths to reduce photosynthetic irradiance in species cultivated in extensive surfaces such as cereals seems unlikely, so a more feasible measure is the management of the soil carbon pool contained in organic matter, which through its transformation by edaphic microbiome is a major source of CO_2 for plants [30].

The soil organic matter results from the transformation of the organic remains of living beings, being an important part the root remains and its exudates. A part of this organic matter is available to be metabolized by soil microorganisms, which produce CO_2 as a by-product. As a consequence, the concentration of CO_2 in the soil pores is very high (1500–6500 $\mu L\ L^{-1}$) and moves through diffusion from the soil to the atmosphere and the canopy of the plants [30]. However, the CO_2 flow rate depends on the organic matter concentration of the soil, which should be managed in the crop fields to values around 5% or more. The use of cover crops and the use of composites, biosolids or biochar incorporated into the soil are ways to increase soil organic matter [31]. Additionally, more organic matter in soil dilute the salts applied with the water and the fertilizers, mitigating the salinization of the soil.

In soils with organic matter at low levels, the process of reaching the adequate concentration of this component of the soil can take years. However, it is possible to achieve the contribution of CO_2 through the soil with the use of humic substances added to the soil. These complex organic compounds provide other advantages such as increasing the availability of minerals to plants, promoting the microbiome of crops and reducing the susceptibility of plants to certain pathogens [31]. The amounts of humic acids used are 5–15 kg ha^{-1}, up to 50–300 kg ha^{-1} [32]; the application can be done using the irrigation system or mixed with fertilizers applied to the soil. In the case of soils with high amounts of calcium carbonate and high pH, the use of strong acids such as H_2SO_4 and HNO_3 (15 L ha^{-1} $week^{-1}$) produces good results, since decreases soil pH and the reaction of acids with carbonates produces CO_2. In addition to strong acids, citric acid (10^{-4} M in nutrient solution or 30–90 kg ha^{-1}) has also been used as well as humic substances [33].

Efficient use of the constant flow of CO_2 from the soil by plants is achieved by using high-density plantings or, in the case of lower density planting, the use of dry straw coverings or other plant debris and the use of plastic mulching that concentrate the flow of the soil CO_2 in the canopy. Maintaining an adequate concentration of CO_2 in the vegetable canopy improves stress tolerance caused by high irradiance [34].

Among the additional advantages of having an adequate amount of organic matter in soil are that it increases the water storage capacity of the soil, increases the availability of mineral elements such as P, S, and Fe, enhances the connectivity between different volumes of the soil which improves the mobility of dissolved minerals [35], a more abundant and more biodiverse microbiome is developed that, among other effects, decreases the susceptibility and the opportunity of invasion by phytopathogenic microorganisms, increases the availability of mineral nutrients of the plants through the association with symbionts and improves plant tolerance to stress through the production of growth regulators, and soluble or volatile metabolites [36].

Soils that have a suitable store of organic matter have the characteristic of behaving like a carbon sink, that is, part of their microbiome can induce the fixation of CO_2 using different metabolic processes. This process seems to establish a balance with the constant loss of CO_2 by microbial respiration [37]. The stability of the soil organic matter store appears to be a characteristic of the ecosystem rather than a chemical characteristic of soil carbon compounds [31], which also points to the importance of maintaining the abundance and biodiversity of the edaphic microbiome, as well as to promote the rotation of crops and the biological diversity of vegetal components in the agricultural ecosystems. Among the processes that have a negative impact on the soil carbon store are photo-oxidation and oxidation induced by excessive tillage, which should be avoided as much as possible. Another factor that negatively affects soil organic matter is a high microbial respiratory rate caused by high diurnal and nocturnal temperatures or by the excessive application of fertilizers with N [38].

3.2. Efficiency of the energy dissipation and redox balance processes

It was explained earlier that when a condition of high irradiance and low availability of CO_2 in the canopy prevails, a considerable part of the solar energy absorbed by the leaf is dissipated by photochemical systems in the form of thermal radiation and free radicals. Energy dissipation products disrupt cellular processes, causing the already mentioned adverse effects such as the decrease in the photosynthetic rate and the oxidative damage of cellular components.

The excess of PAR causes excessive production of reducing potential that is signaled by the redox state of plastoquinone, thioredoxin, and by the generation of ROS, H_2O_2 and $^1O_2$. The perception of these compounds or the byproducts of the interaction of the ROS with membranes and biomolecules, causes modifications in the programs of development directed to the defense against stress causing the synthesis of compounds and antioxidant proteins such as ascorbate, superoxide dismutase, and ascorbate peroxidase, osmolytes, chaperone proteins and in general chemical compounds that signal and combat the resulting oxidative damages such as salicylic acid, ABA, and glutathione [39]. An accumulation of anthocyanins and flavonoids is also present in the vacuole, which can absorb and dissipate excess PAR [40]. The activation of these responses to stress decreases the photosynthetic rate since it reduces the synthesis of proteins related to ATP synthesis and the PSII complex [41].

Different techniques have been proposed for the management of damage caused by high irradiance, among which are the use of genetically modified plants [12], the application of antioxidant compounds, tolerance inducers such as proline and salicylic acid or its derivatives [42], the application of silicon or selenium to the soil or by foliar spraying [43, 44], the maintenance of adequate levels of foliar calcium [45], the use of diverse nanomaterials that besides serving as a nutrient for the plant induce stress tolerance [46], the use of beneficial microorganisms [36], the application of particle-films such as kaolinite which increase foliar reflectance [47, 48] or plant varieties with epidermis with high reflectance such as *glossy* sorghum [49]. As far as it is known, there are no techniques available to induce hardening in plants against high irradiance stress [10].

Regarding the need to have a greater volume of water in the soil, in order to counteract the higher rate of leaf transpiration resulting from the increase in leaf temperature, it was already mentioned that organic matter in the soil increases its storage and water retention capacity, but hydrophilic synthetic materials such as polyacrylamide (20–50 kg ha^{-1}) or polyacrylamide combined with biochar are also available which significantly increase water storage capacity in soil or substrates [50].

Proper plant nutrition is a key factor for plants to have the resources for signaling and defense against stress induced by high irradiance. Adequate nutrition considers, on the one hand, the necessary amounts of nutrients in such a way as to cause excesses or deficiencies and, on the other hand, adequate nutrient balances in such a way that no induced deficiencies are generated. Taking into account that most of the indispensable mineral elements are directly involved in photosynthesis (Mn, Ca, Cl, Fe, Mg) and biochemical reactions (C, N, S, P, K, Ca, Zn, Mg) a key factor in stress management by high irradiance is based on adequate crop nutrition. When high-efficiency irrigation systems are available in soil-less systems, nutrient management can be carried out very precisely, but when the plants are grown in soil, soil characteristics, especially the amount of organic matter and the associated microbiome, regulate the availability of the mineral elements. In the latter case, management of plant nutrition through the management of soil organic matter would promote a resilient edaphic system that allows the mineral elements necessary for plants to be available.

All of the aforementioned techniques have proven useful in mitigating damage caused by high irradiance in plants, but it should not be overlooked that the use of them is directed at the treatment of symptoms, while the primary reason (the combination of high irradiance with little CO_2 in the canopy) is the one that should receive more attention.

On the other hand, it is important to consider that stress due to high irradiance is a characteristic intrinsic to current atmospheric conditions. When the first terrestrial plants made their appearance during the Ordovician, the sun brightness was lower than in the present time, and the CO_2 concentration in the air was 14–22 times greater than the current one [51]. That means that existing plants, with virtually the same photosynthetic systems that originated in bacteria billions of years ago and reconfigured to the present form hundreds of millions of years ago, face a condition where it is practically impossible to avoid saturation by light. However, creating plants that have a better adaptation and response to environmental stressors is not an impossibility [52], but will require a great investment of time, human and material resources, with the support of data science, systems biology, synthetic biology, ecology and soil science, among others.

4. High temperature stress

Currently temperate and subtropical agricultural areas can withstand substantial losses in crop yield due to extreme temperature events [53]. Due to global climate change, a high temperature is projected to be a very relevant abiotic stress factor since it adversely affects plant growth and hence crop yields [54]. Although plants may be more or less resistant to high temperatures depending on the adaptations of each species and geographic location, almost all show a reduction in their growth as a result of unexpected extreme temperature fluctuations [55].

As with high irradiance, stress caused by high temperature can be described at the molecular level or in the cellular or physiological-morphological ambits. In this case, the primary inducing factor is the impact of temperature at the molecular level, which is transferred to other scopes of description such as physiological-morphological interactions between the biomolecules that give rise to different metabolic pathways and activities of cellular metabolism such as energy metabolism and the transport of ions and metabolites. This fact results in the hardening or cross-resistance process being difficult to achieve for stress induced by high temperatures [10].

4.1. Responses at molecular level

From a physical point of view, the temperature is an indicator of the average speed (kinetic energy) of translation or vibration of the molecules that make up the matter. To operate the biochemical reactions biomolecules require a certain temperature to ensure contact with the substrates or receptors with which they interact. This reaction capacity occurs at a very low rate when the temperature falls below a certain threshold (usually 10°C) or occurs at high or excessive rates with temperatures >35°C.

On the other hand, at the molecular level, all the membranes, biomolecules and water associated with these structures have a particular temperature spectrum where the tertiary and quaternary structure of proteins, nucleic acids, and membranes is maintained optimally, as well as the cohesion between biomolecules in multiprotein complexes and protein-nucleic acid complexes. Particularly for the membranes temperature determines an important characteristic known as fluidity, on which the interaction of the integral proteins depends, many of them are sensors or participants in the energy metabolism. However, when it occurs that the thermal vibration exceeds the forces of interaction and cohesion, the result is that the functionality of the biomolecules or their complexes is compromised, initially diminishing their catalytic or functional capacity until they reach inactivation or denaturation when it is exceeded a certain threshold. Similarly, the proteins that are synthesized during the high-temperature period can suffer from misfolding, which makes them non-functional [56]. For terrestrial plants, the threshold where the temperature begins to negatively affect the biomolecules and the processes of interaction between them, is between 35 and 45°C, depending on the specific metabolic activity and the adaptation of each species to a particular environment. For most C3 plants the threshold is at 35°C, whereas C4 species have a response threshold around 40°C. Much of this difference between the two physiological groups is that the solubility of CO_2 declines faster than that of O_2 as the temperature rises, and that RUBISCO shows higher affinity for O_2 at high temperatures [23].

When the temperature exceeds the threshold mentioned above, changes in membrane fluidity, or the lower effectiveness or inactivation of biomolecules associated with electron transport in energy and biosynthetic metabolism, causes the production of ROS in large quantities, leading to oxidative stress. Along with changes in membrane fluidity, ROS production is one of the factors perceived at the molecular level that triggers defense responses against high temperature. It has been observed that acclimatization in plants is possible by exposing them to 5–8°C above the optimal temperature for their growth and development, generating changes in the gene expression associated with the modification of the composition of the membranes, to the production of enzymatic and non-enzymatic antioxidants and osmolytes. For this reason, the exogenous application of some osmolytes and growth regulators such as proline, glycine betaine, salicylic acid, jasmonic acid, IAA, GA, and ABA or the use of sodium selenite is useful in the mitigation of high-temperature stress [57].

Another response at the molecular level triggered by high temperature is the induction of the synthesis of proteins called heat shock (HSPs). These constitute a family of low molecular weight proteins of 15–30 kDa. HSPs accumulate as granular structures in the cytoplasm protecting the mechanisms of protein synthesis [58]. HSPs work by allowing the appropriate post-transcriptional folding of the new proteins or by maintaining the existing proteins in a functional state [56]. Plant cells respond rapidly to high-temperature stress by accumulating HSPs which in turn trigger increased expression of additional genes related to stress mitigation, whose products can act as chaperonins to stabilize proteins by protecting them from denaturation [59]. This fact indicates that it is possible to obtain thermotolerance by stimulating the accumulation of HSPs, either with the use of genetically modified crops or with the application of tolerance inducers such as H_2O_2 and salicylic acid [60].

Another alternative for handling high-temperature stress in field crops is the use of chemical elements in the nanometric form. The application of $nTiO_2$ [61], CeO_2 [62], and nSe [63], demonstrated effectiveness in inducing protection against stress caused by high temperature. Given the complexity of managing this stress and the projection that it will be increasingly common, the use of nanomaterials deserves further exploration.

4.2. Responses at the cellular and physiological-morphological level

Metabolic processes such as photosynthesis, respiration, transpiration, absorption, transport and assimilation of nutrients, among others, also have temperature spectra for their proper functioning. These responses depend in part on the phenomena described for the molecular domain, but also on the interactions between the biomolecules and their complexes that form the different metabolic pathways, as well as on the interactions between the different metabolic pathways that produce precursor compounds or which are source and information for other metabolic pathways.

In the scale of the interaction of the plant structures with the canopy atmosphere, the high temperature causes a very high vapor pressure deficit, which results in high foliar transpiration that competes with the flow of water to other organs such as flowers and fruits, especially when the high temperature also occurs at night time. When transpiration (cooling) capacity is exceeded by the absorption of solar radiation (heating), a condition that occurs most quickly with high irradiance and air temperature >35°C, burns occur on leaves, stems, and fruits, senescence and foliar abscission, inhibition of growth and root damage affecting nutrient uptake, resulting in low yield and poor quality [64]. On the other hand, high temperatures decrease the viability of pollen [65] and shorten the period in which stigmas in flowers are receptive to pollen, reducing the chances of successful fertilization [66].

As mentioned, photosynthesis is more affected in C3 plants than in C4 plants due to the high temperature, and again the concentration of CO_2 in the canopy is an important factor to mitigate the damage caused by high temperatures. The higher concentration of CO_2 allows to reduce photorespiration and increase the photosynthetic rate, decrease transpiration and increase the production of antioxidants in the leaves [67]. The higher concentration of CO_2 in the canopy of the plants, associated with the maintenance or increase in soil organic matter, appears again as a multifunctional tool for the management of stress [68]. For the mitigation of damages by high temperature, it is also useful to apply hydrophilic polymers, incorporating these materials into the soil or substrate increases the water retention and storage capacity, decreasing the rate of evaporation loss that accompanies the high temperature. As a consequence, more water is available to be absorbed by plants [69].

On the other hand, the presence of microorganisms associated with soil organic matter has also been found as a factor promoting tolerance to high-temperature stress in plants [70]. Different fungi that form arbuscular mycorrhiza have been shown to be useful in the mitigation of damages induced by high temperature, both by increasing the production of antioxidant metabolites and the activity of antioxidant enzymes, as well as allowing a better response in photosynthesis and water use efficiency in crops [71, 72].

As we have seen, there is a high amount of work that describes the adjustments made by plants against heat, both at the molecular level with studies in the transcriptome and proteome as well as in the metabolic and physiological field with biochemical studies of specific metabolic pathways, physiological studies of photosynthesis, respiration and growth [56, 57]. However, an important aspect to which less attention is given is that in other scopes of description, for example in ecosystems the high temperatures also impose modifications in the interactions of its components, causing changes in the structure and dynamics, it is still poorly understood and difficult to predict [73].

5. Low temperature stress

Low-temperature stress is an environmental factor that greatly affects the growth, development, and productivity of plants. This type of environmental stress includes non-freezing temperatures (0°C < T < 10°C) as well as freezing temperatures (T < 0°C). Crop plants originating in the tropics or subtropics die or are severely damaged when exposed to low freezing temperatures, even for short periods (24–48 hours), developing symptoms such as chlorosis, necrosis or stunting. In contrast, species originated from temperate and subarctic zones through an adaptive process that develops during the fall can tolerate freezing temperatures [74]. However, although different species of plants may be more or less resistant to low temperatures depending on the adaptations of each species and their origin or geographical location, they all show a reduction in growth against unexpected events of low temperature as the unexpected nature of the phenomenon does not allow the natural adaptive process to begin [15].

The stress caused by low temperature can be described at the molecular level or in the cellular or physiological-morphological ambits. The primary inducing factor is the impact of low temperature on the reduction of the speed of vibration and translation of the molecules (in the presence of low temperatures) and the total deficit or absence of water when it becomes ice when there are freezing temperatures. Such changes are transferred to other levels of description such as physiological-morphological interactions between biomolecules that give rise to different metabolic pathways and cellular activities such as energy metabolism and transport of ions and metabolites. This fact results in that the process of hardening or cross-resistance (with the exception for the damages caused by the oxidative stress) is difficult to achieve for the stress induced by the low temperatures, especially when they cause freezing [15].

5.1. Responses at the molecular level

From a physical point of view the low non-freezing temperature has an impact contrary to that described for the high temperature because it decreases the speed of vibration of the molecules; in membranes reduces the average distance between molecules and decreases fluidity. This change in fluidity considerably modifies the behavior of integral proteins, many of which are associated with energy metabolism. The result is the production of ROS and consequent oxidative stress [15]. It has been hypothesized that the decrease in membrane fluidity is the primary site of low-temperature stress perception [75] and it has been found that one of the first adaptive responses of cells increases the lipid unsaturation of the membranes, which increases their fluidity [76]. After the initial perception of changes in membrane fluidity, Ca^{2+} fuses from the apoplast and vacuole stores are triggered into the cytoplasm [77]. Calcium fluxes activate MAPK cascades that result in changes in the activity of transcription factors that initiate an extensive network of transcriptional, posttranscriptional, and posttranslational responses involving more than 2000 genes associated with low-temperature responses [78]. Therefore, maintaining the proper nutritional status of plants, especially concerning calcium concentration in different organs, is critical to ensure an adequate response to changes in temperature.

In mitochondria, the low temperature causes a slower rate of consumption of the reducing potential, which results in the production of ROS and the activation of a specialized enzyme called mitochondrial alternative oxidase (chloroplasts also have an alternative oxidase). The mitochondrial alternative oxidase is an indicator of the plant response to low temperature, allowing the dissipation of reducing potential to transform it into heat and reduce the formation of ROS. The mitochondrial alternative oxidase can be activated through exogenous applications of salicylic acid and was demonstrated to work by mitigating oxidative stress in mitochondria against other stresses [79].

The low temperature also causes the elevation of the activation energy of the biochemical reactions, modifying the interactions between the multitude of enzymes and proteins associated with cellular energy processes. Each metabolic pathway is affected differently by low temperature, but the result is an imbalance in the generation and use of energy, which causes oxidative stress and less energy availability for cell growth and maintenance. Among the measures used to mitigate the damage of stress by low temperatures is the exogenous application of tolerance inducers such as salicylic acid, beneficial elements such as silicon and various nanomaterials [79–81], application of osmolytes such as glycine betaine and proline [82], or the use of genetically modified crops with a higher synthesis capacity of these compounds [12].

It has also been determined that phytohormones play a major role in the induction of tolerance at low temperatures. Hormones create a complex network of interactions that are used to integrate external information into endogenous development programs and activate the stress response pathways that lead to resistance. The knowledge of hormone regulatory activities against low temperature is limited, although it is known that they are involved in signaling cascades of other types of biotic and abiotic stress [83].

The stress induced by freezing is different from that caused by low temperature. When freezing of plant tissues occurs, this begins in the apoplast, which is the volume of water that is in contact with the external surfaces of leaves, stems, flowers, and fruits. Typically the freezing process takes place outside the plant toward the interior of the plant and is accelerated by the presence of dust and microorganisms that function as seeds for the formation of the first ice crystals. The presence of mechanical damage (hail, wind) or biotic (pests or pathogens) increases the possibility of contact between the water from the exterior and the interior of the plant and therefore are factors that facilitate freezing. Once the water from the apoplast begins to freeze at some point, the process spreads rapidly to the rest of the plant. The disappearance of water caused by the formation of ice causes a severe water deficit that causes a rapid denaturation of cellular components and cell death [84]. The damage caused by freezing is very different from that induced by the low temperature and makes it extremely complicated regarding its control or genetic improvement of crops.

5.2. Responses at the cellular and physiological-morphological level

The metabolic processes dependent on biochemical reactions are affected by the low temperature more rapidly than the photochemical processes. The presence of PAR aggravates the induced damages by low temperature, and the plants are quickly photo-inhibited, the reason why some of the measures described to mitigate the damage by high irradiance are applicable for low temperature. It has been found that the photo-inhibition process is also present when low temperatures occur at night, this adjustment is thought to be part of the adaptive response to low temperature [85]. Photosynthesis is affected to a large extent, the cessation of growth reduces the capacity of energy utilization, with the consequent production of ROS and oxidative stress [86].

Many antioxidant enzymes are involved in low-temperature response machinery. In addition to those associated with the metabolism of osmolytes, detoxification cascades and photosynthesis, the metabolism of lignin (caffeic acid 3-O-methyltransferase), secondary metabolism, remodeling of cell wall polysaccharides, metabolism of starch, sterol biosynthesis and the oligosaccharide of the raffinose family (myoinositol-phosphate synthase and galactinol synthase) are all participants in the overall response to cold stress [87, 88].

Carbohydrates, mainly sucrose, function as osmolytes and antioxidants to protect cells and their components against oxidative damage. A high value of CO_2 in the canopy of plants is associated with higher amounts of carbohydrates in different plant structures [89]. Soil organic matter, as a source of CO_2 for plants, and as a factor to increase soil fertility and magnitude and diversity of the plant microbiome, may be a factor to mitigate damage against cold stress [90, 91]. An additional advantage of organic matter in soil is to increase the water storage capacity, as the thermal capability of the water is much greater than that of the air so a soil with a substantial volume of water will be able to store heat that will radiate to the plants during the night or a low-temperature period or frost event.

6. Water stress

The available water for crop plants is located in two storages: the edaphic and the atmospheric. The atmospheric storage includes water that precipitates as rain, dew, mist, or snow, in addition to the water contained in the air in the form of water vapor and, together with temperature, determines the vapor pressure deficit (VPD). VPD is strongly associated with stomatal responses and therefore has an impact on photosynthesis and productivity [68].

VPD and water in the atmosphere are difficult to control in open field since they depend on the weather stations, prevailing winds, topography, surrounding vegetation, the presence of nearby bodies of water, etc. On the other hand, according to the models of climate change, the forecast of the availability of atmospheric water will be more and more complicated, and it is expected that the crops in the open field are exposed with increasing frequency and intensity to periods of shortage of atmospheric water [92], this projection is, however, subject to discussion because of the opposite effect that could exert the increase in atmospheric CO_2 on carbon transpiration and metabolism in forest species [93].

The structure and functionality of biomolecules, membranes, and cytoskeleton, the availability of electrons and protons during photosynthesis, the solubility of gases such as CO_2 and mineral ions depend on water [94]. The plants perceive the water deficit through stimuli related to the different functions the water carries out. These include: (a) stabilization of the functional form of proteins, nucleic acids, lipids of membranes, and in general of the different biomolecules and ions with which metabolism occurs; (b) water is a biochemical and electrochemical source for organisms, contributing H^+ and e^- which are used in energy metabolism, as well as in antioxidant metabolism related to productivity, adaptation to the environment and in the development and differentiation; (c) the provision of mechanical support for stems, leaves, flowers, and fruits; (d) the transpiration process for the maintenance of temperature during the absorption of electromagnetic radiation [14].

6.1. Responses at the molecular level

As with high-temperature stress, the water deficit causes the loss of structure and functionality of the biomolecules, creating a general imbalance in the energy metabolism that results in the formation of ROS and oxidative damage to the cellular structures. These oxidative damages are increased in the presence of high irradiance and high temperature, a combination of stresses that is expected to become increasingly common [10].

At the molecular level the response of the plant to this type of stress comes in three forms: the first is to induce the synthesis of antioxidants and chaperone proteins to eliminate ROS and preserve the structure of other biomolecules; the second is the synthesis of osmolytes that function as antioxidants as well as differential exclusion agents that stabilize membranes, proteins, and nucleic acids under water deficit conditions. The same osmolytes serve as a source of N and C to recover cell growth when the stress condition decreases; the third is to increase the rate of degradation of proteins that have undergone oxidative damage or that have aberrant folds, the latter is a response that eliminates non-functional biomolecules and in addition, allows to recover amino acids that can be used for synthesis of other proteins or as a source of C y N in other metabolic pathways [95, 96].

The set of cellular metabolic processes are related to each other through energy signals that constitute redox balance, as well as exchanges of molecules that are products of a particular metabolic pathway, and in others function as regulators or effectors. For this reason, all metabolic processes are sensitive to water deficit, although the level of sensitivity is variable among them [95]. As explained in the Introduction, many of the responses to stress have a direct impact on energy metabolism because it depends on many integral membrane enzymes that are particularly susceptible to loss of functionality due to lack of water or changes in the temperature. Therefore, many of the studies on the induction of tolerance to water deficit refer to the energy metabolism, in particular to the oxidative stress resulting from the imbalances between the supply of reducing potential and ATP and its use in the processes that function as energy sinks.

If it is sought to reduce the damage that occurs in plants against the water deficit, it can be achieved by the exogenous application antioxidant compounds, osmolytes, growth regulators such as ABA, IAA, and GA [97, 98], tolerance inducers such as salicylates and other organic acids or amino acids [79]. Their use in specific situations will depend on the application opportunity, the cost and the application capacities in the particular crop in question. On the other hand, for compounds that individually exert a positive effect by increasing tolerance to stress, it is also feasible to produce transgenic crops with advantages over their wild counterparts [12].

With this information, it can be concluded that, at the biochemical and metabolic level, the opportunities to mitigate the damage to plants against the water deficit are broad, but again they should be framed in a comprehensive effort that considers soil, irrigation management, and planting systems, among others.

6.2. Responses at the cellular and physiological-morphological level

Transpiration is the most important component of water use by plants regarding volume. A typical wheat or corn crop requires 453 and 423 mm per season in the absence of water stress. Of this amount of water, 70% corresponds to transpiration [99]. Unless the temperature or the irradiance is reduced, the light interception is reduced, or the leaf albedo is increased, it is challenging to decrease the transpiration rate since the heat dissipation obtained through the transpiration avoids damages by high temperature in foliar metabolic components, especially those involved in photosynthesis, while on the other hand the decrease in stomatal conductance required to reduce transpiration would lead to a lower photosynthetic rate [68]. It was already mentioned in the subchapter dedicated to high irradiance stress the use of techniques such as increasing soil organic matter to release more CO_2 in the canopy, thus increasing water use efficiency, use of kaolinite as an anti-transpirant and reflector for increase leaf albedo, genetic selection of glossy varieties or to obtain plants with higher density of trichomes and a consequent greater leaf albedo. These same techniques are used to mitigate the water deficit in crops.

On the other hand water acts as a medium that provides mechanical support to herbaceous plants and photosynthetic and reproductive organs of shrub and tree plants, this is achieved by transporting water to the cells and apoplast to maintain cellular turgor. The water deficit causes loss of turgor that is perceived through mechanoreceptors that trigger part of the stress signaling pathways and ultimately cause the loss of green tissues [100]. The higher tolerance to turgidity loss is associated with changes in the composition and structure of the polymers of the cell wall, or due to the particular composition of the cell walls, as well as the ability to retain water in the vacuole and in the apoplast against the low water potential in the apoplast by modifying aquaporin density and activity [101]. In this sense, this characteristic of turgor retention is complex from the genomic, biochemical, metabolic, and structural perspective; is different between ecotypes or varieties of the same species, obtaining the differences through natural selection or genetic selection. Therefore its manipulation corresponds to techniques of plant genetics and transgenic crops [12]. During the induction of water stress, this process of turgor loss and loss of photosynthetic tissues is the last to occur, since it is preceded by the responses associated with the decrease in productive metabolism and growth.

One way to mitigate the adverse effect of a high VPD in a field is to increase the concentration of CO_2 in the canopy of plants, as more elevated [CO_2] results in an increase in photosynthetic capacity, including partial closure of the stomata which decreases the water vapor loss of the mesophyll [68]. It is known that a greater amount of OM in the soil and the planting of high density crops allow higher [CO_2] and decrease of evaporation in the soil, in addition to the buffer effect on the loss of moisture in the canopy by wind and convective processes caused by the proximity of other plants [30, 92].

In practical terms, the edaphic water storage is the one within reach for manipulation and control in agricultural production systems. The water absorption and retention capacity of the soil depend on the set of forces between the components of the water potential:

$$\Psi = \Psi_g + \Psi_p + \Psi_o + \Psi_m \tag{1}$$

The losses due to leaching (Ψ_g) and evapotranspiration of the soil and plants are in dynamic balance with the components that allow the conservation of the water, which are the matric or capillary potential (Ψ_m) and the osmotic potential (Ψ_o), which refer to the molecular interactions between water and the structural components (such as soil pores), physicochemical (inorganic colloids) and biological (organic colloids) of the soil, as well as the ions dissolved in the water of the soil pores. These interactions occur at different scales, from nanometric to micrometric.

The practical way to maintain or increase ability of the soil to absorb and conserve water in the edaphic profile accessible to crop plants (0.1–1.5 m) has been described with different techniques of rainwater harvesting [102] and soil conservation, among which we can mention low tillage to conserve soil pore structure and the use of cover crops [103], the promotion of beneficial microorganisms in the soil [70] and the use of hydrophilic polymers. A relatively simple way to increase the soil ability to provide water to crops at medium and long term is to increase the amount of organic matter, which increases the soil matric potential. Different reports indicate the direct relationship between a higher concentration of organic matter, higher water retention capacity, and plant response in the form of less impact on growth when irrigation water or atmospheric precipitation is reduced [104]. In that sense, any strategy aimed at raising crop tolerance to water deficits under the current climate change scenario must take into account the increase in soil organic matter as well as the counterpart of its biological activity [70].

The use of grafts, although applied almost exclusively to horticultural species, offers good results mitigating damage by different stresses, mainly high temperature, salinity, water deficit, and root pathogens [105]. On the other hand, the use of fertilizers with silicon (Na_2SiO_3 200–800 kg ha^{-1} to the soil or 123 mg L^{-1} in the nutrient solution), selenium (10 g ha^{-1} to the soil or 0.5–3.0 mg L^{-1} by foliar spraying), or selenium and sulfur (as elemental sulfur S0, applying 20–80 kg ha^{-1} to the soil) decreases the negative responses of the plant to the water deficit. Although the mechanisms that explain the benefits of these elements in plants are still not well understood, their use has repeatedly been reported obtaining satisfactory results [106–108]. Both silicon and selenium, and sulfur can induce hardening in plants again stress caused by water deficit.

An effective alternative, although rarely used in field crops because of its high cost, is the application in furrows or seed beds, of biodegradable hydrophilic polymers such as single polyacrylamide (25–100 kg ha^{-1}) or in combination with biochar [69]. Polyacrylamide has a shelf life of 3 years once it is applied to the soil and can absorb 100 or more times its weight in water, conserving the water in its molecular structure against leaching and evaporation processes. The effectiveness of hydrophilic polymers depends on the salinity of the water, being ineffective with electrical conductivities higher than 4000 $\mu S\ cm^{-1}$ or with calcium-rich water [109]. Other techniques used in the field such as the use of natural or plastic mulching and the application of water using drip irrigation systems are also potentially useful as a means of increasing the efficiency of water use [110]. The use of the different techniques mentioned, using an integrated approach to improve the absorption and conservation of soil water, is the best recommendation.

7. Salinity stress

Until a few decades ago the cultivation in saline soils was not considered as an alternative for food, fiber, or biomass production. However, the stress induced by the presence of large amounts of salts in soils and water has taken on current importance due to the progressive salinization of agricultural soils, resulting in the extraction of water from the subsoil, the higher evapotranspiration resulting from the increase in temperatures and by rainfall regimes, which occur more erratically. Along with the gradual loss of organic matter from soils, salinization is considered an increasingly common symptom of soil degradation [111, 112].

The first step to cultivate in saline or salinization soil due to the use of irrigation water in combination with high evapotranspiration is to determine whether the crop will be destined to produce food, fiber, or biomass. The point is important because it is more feasible to find a species with some tolerance to salinity to produce fiber or biomass (which could later be transformed into biofuel) than one for the production of food such as corn, wheat, or tomato. Part of the strategy to achieve greater agricultural production in saline or salinized soils is perhaps to correctly select the plant species to be cultivated in such a way that the natural abilities of the different plant species are part of the solution to the growing problem of salinity in agricultural systems. As has been said for other stresses, there is an intrinsic incompatibility between high productivity and high yields and stress tolerance, since both processes depend on the same budget of photosynthates for successful development. The case of salinity is complex regarding its management and the obtaining of improved varieties since it involves two stresses in one: osmotic and ionic, affecting many different aspects of the growth, development, physiology, and biochemistry of plants (**Figure 2**).

A relevant part of the solution is to give greater attention to halophytic species, both as a source of genetic resources to improve glycophytic crops, and for direct use in the rehabilitation processes of salinized soils or for cultivation in saline soils seeking to produce fodder, pigments, or biomass for industrial processing, seems to be of increasing importance [113].

7.1. Responses at the molecular level

Salinity-induced stress occurs in two phases: the first occurs very rapidly (the plant's perception takes place in in seconds and the signaling and response in minutes or hours) and is a result of the decrease in the water potential of soil pore water or nutrient solution by the high concentration of dissolved ions present. The low water potential makes it difficult for water to be absorbed by the roots and a water deficit is induced, with signaling and responses as described in the previous Section of Water Stress, including decreased growth, ABA synthesis, and stomatal closure [114]. The second phase occurs at a later time to the first and is a result of the gradual intoxication of the cells mainly by Na^+ and Cl^-, which interfere with the ionic balance in the cytoplasm that depends mostly on K^+, Mg^{2+} and NO_3^- [115].

At the molecular level, there are three defense mechanisms of the plant against the high concentration of salts in the soil solution or nutrient solution: (i) osmotic tolerance and root exclusion, (ii) osmotic tolerance and foliar exclusion, and (iii) Na^+ tolerance. The first mechanism depends on the interruption of the production of radical hairs and new leaves, stomatal closure, and increased root growth toward new soil volumes. Root exclusion depends on the control of Na^+ and Cl^- flux in the endodermis (which depends significantly on the availability of silicon). However, as Na^+ and Cl^- enter the cytoplasm via nonselective channels and transporters, it is inevitable that they will reach the xylem and thence to the rest of the plant [111, 115, 116]. An important part of the osmotic response in the root is based on the increase in aquaporin density in the cells of the epidermis; it is believed that this response improves the water status of the root [116].

When the first root exclusion mechanism fails, Na^+ and Cl^- accumulate in stem and leaf apoplast, activating a foliar osmotic tolerance response that depends on the synthesis of enzymatic and non-enzymatic antioxidants, to counteract the most of ROS production, and synthesis of osmolytes such as proline, polyols, and glycine betaine to preserve the functionality of membranes, proteins, and other biomolecules. On the other hand, Na^+ and Cl^- of the apoplast are transported to the cytoplasm of the cells by means of nonspecific channels and the Na^+/Ca^{2+}, Na^+/K^+, Ca^{2+}/Mg^{2+}, and Cl^-/NO_3^- ionic balance breaks, which interferes with

http://dx.doi.org/10.5772/intechopen.71771

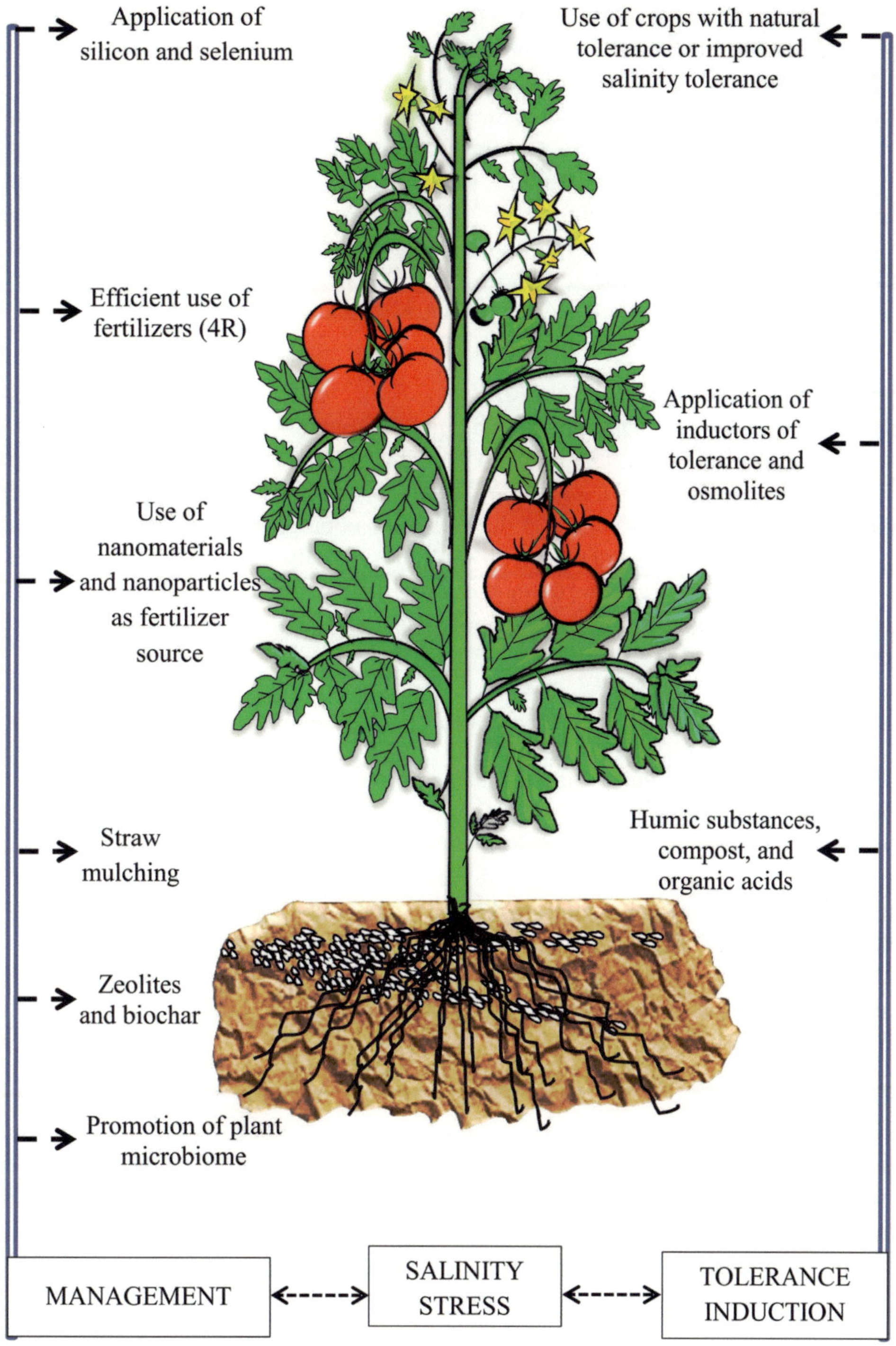

Figure 2. Environmental factors and agronomic management to be used for agricultural production in soils or substrates with high amounts of salts.

the membrane's charge balance on which the activity of the integral proteins depends, and also competitively inhibits a large number of enzymes which are activated by K^+, Mg^{2+} and Ca^{2+}. Plant cells turns on an exclusion process dependent on the pumping of toxic ions to mitigate the accumulation of Na^+. An example of such mechanisms is the SOS proteins that are responsible for transporting the Na^+ from the cytoplasm to the vacuole or the apoplast and is even associated with long-distance transport of Na^+ [112]. These toxic ion-pumping systems, however, have a very high-energy expenditure. As salinity significantly interferes with metabolic processes, the energy budget is getting lower, and over time the cells ability to keep toxic ions out of the cytoplasm volume is exceeded. Then the point where the concentration of Na^+ and Cl^- in the cytoplasm grows in such a way that it causes the death of the cells.

Crops are not very tolerant to Na^+ and Cl^-, but this character is variable from one species to another. Tolerance capacity can be increased if plants have enough Ca^{2+}, K^+, Mg^{2+}, and NO_3^- to mitigate the imbalances caused by Na^+ and Cl^-. Also, the use of antioxidants and osmolytes such as proline and glycine betaine applied exogenously, or the use of enhanced or genetically modified varieties may be useful during the osmotic phase of salinity-induced stress [111, 114]. However, obtaining crops with high productivity and halophytic character is a challenge, since the exclusion, compartmentalization, and extrusion of Na^+ and other ions that reach toxic concentrations requires a high-energy expenditure and therefore a high percentage of the photosynthates produced.

7.2. Responses at the cellular and physiological-morphological level

The osmotic and toxicity effects on the molecular scale are transferred to the upper levels, causing a rapid stomatal closure dependent on ABA, decreased photosynthesis and interruption of growth in young leaves, which is the first symptom observed in the plant. In case the adaptive response is successful, the growth can be restarted at a later time, once the adjustments in the cellular development programs that allow the osmotic tolerance and the Na^+ tolerance occur. If the mechanisms mentioned above of osmotic balance and exclusion are not sufficient, the plant will initiate a gradual process of intoxication characterized by the senescence of mature leaves, a result of the accumulation of Na^+ and Cl^- [111].

7.3. Management of salinity-induced stress

As the primary factor that induces stress is the high concentration of salts in the soil or substrate, stress mitigation is mainly directed to the application of soil management techniques. However, the use of tolerance-inducing compounds such as salicylic acid, antioxidants, osmolytes and growth regulators applied by foliar spraying or in seedlings or seeds, are useful for improving plant response. Also, the use of genetically improved plants is an alternative that can be combined with soil management to obtain better results [112].

From an agronomic perspective, salinity is expressed in terms of electrical conductivity (EC) in units of $dS\ m^{-1}$ ($1\ dS\ m^{-1} = 1000\ \mu S\ cm^{-1}$) or $mmhos\ cm^{-1}$ (equivalent to $1\ dS\ m^{-1}$ or $1\ mS\ cm^{-1}$)

It is usually determined on a saturated past extract soil:water (ECe), in soil taken from the root region of the plant and averaged over depth and time. The ECe of a saturation extract for a heavy soil or medium texture multiplied by 2 marks the approximate EC for soil solution at field capacity. In contrast, for sandy soils, ECe is multiplied by 3. For direct determination in field or greenhouse, filtered extracts of soil:water in relation 1:1, 1:2 or 1:5 volume/volume are used. EC and osmotic potential are linearly related (1 mS cm^{-1} = −0.036 Mpa). The productivity of salinity-sensitive plants decreases if soil EC exceeds 4 mS cm^{-1} (4000 μS cm^{-1}) therefore it is recommended that irrigation water does not exceed 2 mS cm^{-1} [13].

There are several physical-chemical techniques for the management of saline soil conditions that favor crop yields. When soil salinity is not intrinsic but results from the application of fertilizer or irrigation water with high EC, soil management techniques can be used such as drainage improvement and leaching practices, with or without gypsum applications, limestone, and sulfuric acid, as well as deep tillage, subsoiling, and inversion of the soil profile. Several factors, such as the availability of water, the quality of the water, the access to the machinery and the necessary economic resources must be considered before applying the methods above mentioned. The application of localized organic matter (used on rows or seed beds) or throughout the complete soil profile is also useful as a technique to dilute the concentration of salts in the soil explored by the root. This latter technique is also useful when soils are inherently saline [117].

Other methods that mitigate salinity are the incorporation of crop residues, as well as crop rotation and the application of biosolids and biochar to dilute ion concentration in soil and to promote plant microbiome, the latter has been shown to have a positive effect on plants subjected to high salt concentration either by the production of growth hormones, osmolytes and other stress relieving compounds, or because the microorganisms themselves capture part of the salts present and sequester them in their biomolecules over a period. The greater amount of organic matter increases the availability of CO_2, which, even under conditions of partial closure of the stomata, allows the maintenance of photosynthesis, which in turn is associated with greater availability of energy and biomolecules such as antioxidants and osmolytes [117, 118].

On the other hand, an adequate regulation of the nutrients in plants can improve the acclimatization to the saline environment. Application to the soil of silicon fertilizers has shown to be an effective technique to improve tolerance to salinity in plants. The contribution of other mineral nutrients such as K and Ca combined with compost or other sources of organic matter reduces Na^+ absorption, increases K^+ and improves the K^+:Na^+ balance, resulting in higher plant growth and yield. The use of nanofertilizers, which has been shown to be more efficient to feed plants compared to traditional fertilizers [46], could be another alternative to reduce the supply of salts to agricultural soils, thus decreasing the process of salinization that every day increases the surface of degraded soils. Another suitable alternative to mitigate this type of stress is the application of zeolite and humic substances that capture the salts in the soil, reducing the EC of the soil solution, increasing the growth of the roots as well as the uptake of other mineral elements [119, 120].

8. Nutrient deficiency stress

In the other types of stress reviewed, high irradiance, extremes of temperature, water deficit, and salinity, it was explained how the proper management and care of the soil constitutes a critical component for its mitigation. In the case of the deficit of mineral nutrients, this part is especially relevant since the soil or substrate is the primary source of nutrients. Environmental conditions that induce mineral deficiency are manifold, as well as the ability of plant species and their microbiome to absorb, transport, assimilate and store nutrients. The different combinations of irradiance, temperature, relative humidity, physicochemical and biotic characteristics of the soil impose different needs both in quantity and in the molar balance of the elements used by the plants for their metabolism. It is known about C/N, N/P, K/Ca, Ca/Mg, among other ratios, but it is a complex challenge to have the necessary information to appropriately manage the nutrition (time, quantity, chemical form and balance with other elements) of crops during their growth, especially in extensive crops and those developed in the soil.

Different agronomic approaches, such as the 4R and Integrated Nutrient Management (INM), are currently being used to increase the ratio between the amount of fertilizer absorbed by the plants and the amount of fertilizer applied to the soil, or nutrient use efficiency (NUE). The aim is to reduce the ecological and economic costs of agricultural practices, achieving a higher return concerning food production without contravening the sustainability of the edaphic system [103, 121, 122]. The main characteristic of the 4R and INM approaches is that they are integrated processes, not directed to a single practice or a single component of the ecosystem (**Figure 3**).

Almost all of the above practices focus to a greater or lesser extent on soil quality care, quality being defined as soil capacity to provide the environmental services associated with the water cycle and mineral elements, soil support vegetation, animal life and edaphic microbiome, storage of C and other minerals, among others. Soil quality can be monitored in a variety of ways, but a very sensitive indicator is the amount of organic matter in the soil, which, when it decreases, signals a degradation process [103]. The quality of the soil is closely related to the quantity and frequency of tillage applied; the greater the amount of heavy machinery working in the field the greater is the soil degradation.

Another indicator of soil quality is the ability to maintain the necessary mineral elements in a bio-available form for plants. The plants take up through the roots the dissolved elements in the solution of the soil, in turn, this edaphic component is in a homeostatic process of exchange of elements with the mineral and organic components of the soil [124]. The edaphic microbiome plays a key role in this dynamic equilibrium by solubilizing, precipitating and synthesizing new minerals from the available elements. For all the processes before mentioned certain conditions of pH, EC, and redox potential are necessary to facilitate the interchange of elements between the different phases of the system, the organic matter of the soil fulfilling a crucial role in the maintenance of such conditions. Again, as in the stresses described in earlier parts of this manuscript, the importance of conserving and managing organic matter in agricultural soils arises.

http://dx.doi.org/10.5772/intechopen.71771

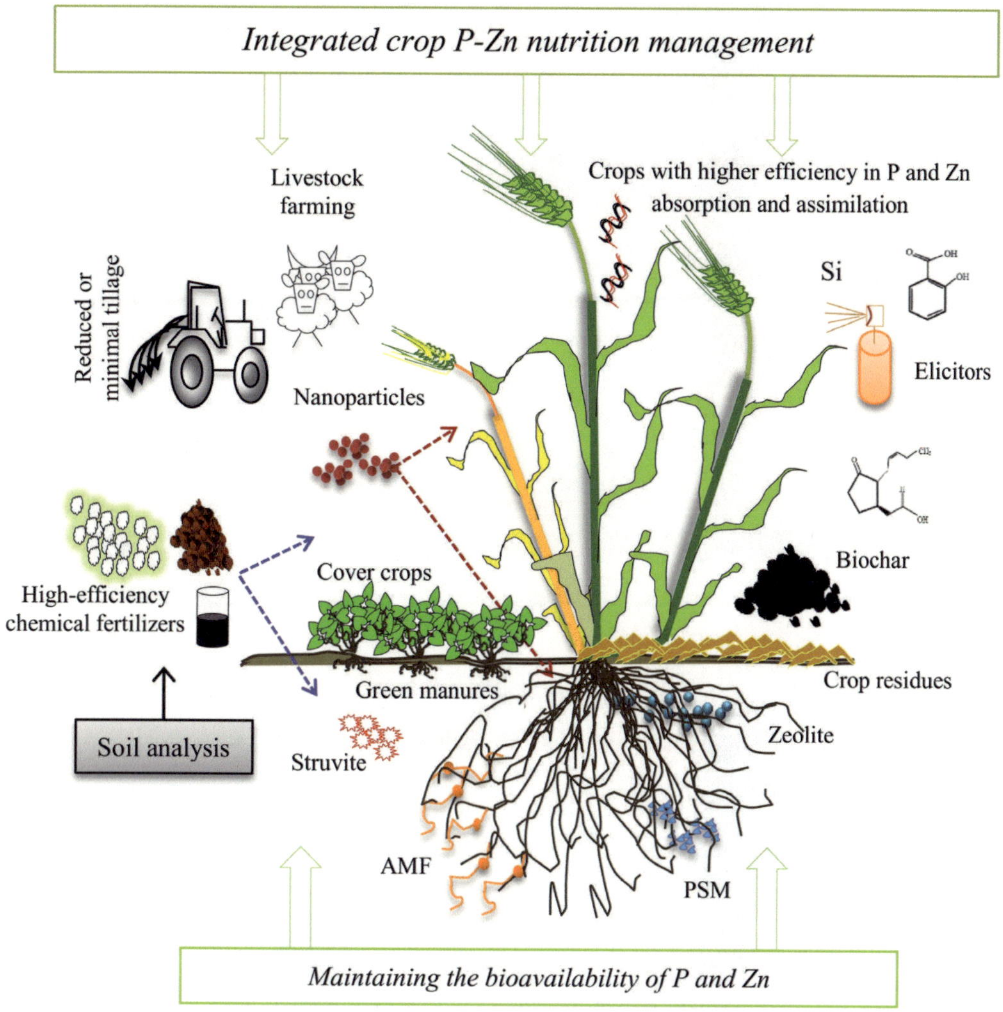

Figure 3. An integrated approach to agronomic practices to mitigate P and Zn deficits in crops. It is an example of the integral agronomic management described in the text, aimed at reducing the deficit of two very relevant nutrients from a perspective of sustainable agricultural production and from the point of view of human food, for which there are restrictions as far as the availability and effectiveness of available fertilizer sources [123].

For most of the mineral elements, high and low-affinity transporters responsible for their absorption, transport to the radical cortex and vascular bundles have been described for their distribution and assimilation in all organs of the plant [125]. The functionality of these transporters depends on the bioavailability of the element in the rhizosphere (the volume of soil modified directly by the root surface). This bioavailability depends on physicochemical factors, which are significantly buffered by the presence of organic matter [122], and biotic factors that encompass the root microbiome and the root activity that modifies the rhizosphere through excretion of organic acids, metabolites, and enzymes, and H^+ that solubilize minerals [126].

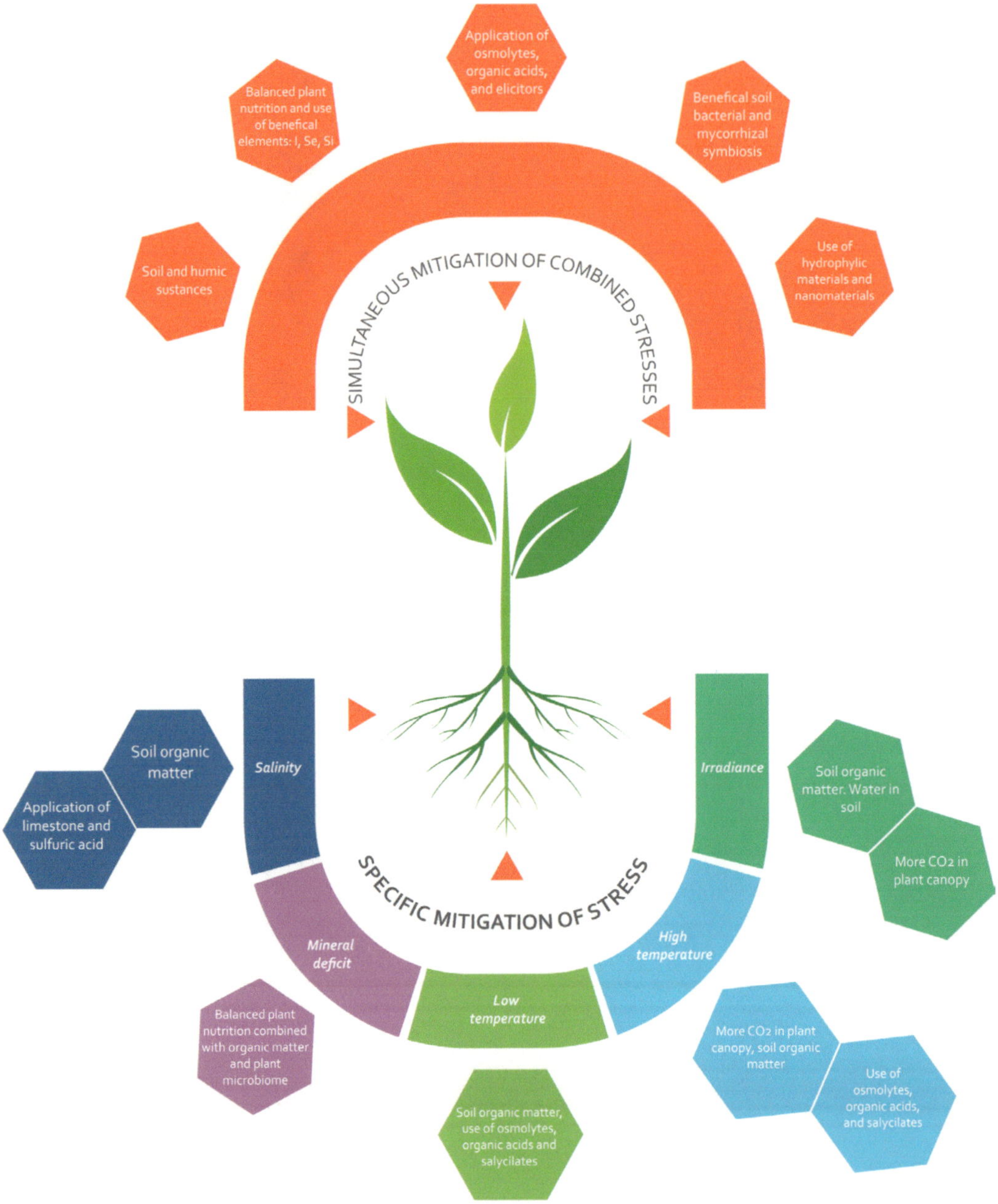

Figure 4. Integral application of different technologies for the management of abiotic stress as a tool to improve food production in a climate change scenario.

The use of cover crops, the incorporation of organic matter in the form of compost, biochar, and biosolids is recommended to increase the bioavailability of mineral elements. In the same way the controlled use of organic and inorganic forms of the applied elements, including the use of rock dust, materials obtained as an industrial by-product, and in the form of nanomaterials, which raises the possibility that the biotic processes and abiotic systems of the soil system transform these materials into nutrients in available forms. Similarly, the application of so-called biological fertilizers or biofertilizers, such as *Rhizobiaceae, Azotobacter, Azospirillum,* vesicular-arbuscular mycorrhizae (VAM), phosphate solubilizing bacteria (PSB), and plant growth-promoting rhizobacteria can be used in combination with organic and inorganic fertilizers [127].

The option of using biofertilizers should be emphasized. Some advantages mean that the alternative of using biofertilizers can be considered as useful to make food production more efficient and sustainable: they are a natural and non-polluting source of fertilizing elements for crops; beneficial microorganisms can be isolated and produced locally, with techniques and technology available in many parts of the world, which also has a multiplier effect of local bio-industries; microorganisms that benefit the plant with a greater bioavailability of mineral elements also increase their productivity and tolerance to abiotic stress through the production of growth regulators and metabolites that restrict the growth of pathogens [128].

Also, the development of nanofertilizers with a greater efficiency in its absorption and impact in the plant is an open subject, but that undoubtedly will contribute of relevant form to the improvement of the nutrition of the plants. It has been proven experimentally that all essential elements for plants are absorbed and used by plants in their nanometric form. However, the more diversified and larger application of this technology still requires that the safety issues of the use of nanomaterials in crops destined to food production be solved [46].

The combination of technologies in an integral way (**Figure 4**) can offer many advantages against a non-benign climate scenario. The greater or lesser bioavailability of mineral elements can be modified through soil improvement practices such as the use of organic matter and the application of inorganic fertilizers and biofertilizers. Soil management and nutrition in combination with the use of crop varieties with greater efficiency in nutrient absorption is also advisable. To do this, from the use of traditional selection techniques to the use of genetically modified varieties or genome-editing are a determining factor in an integrated approach to the management of nutrient deficiencies in agriculture. [129, 130].

9. Conclusions

A comprehensive approach to the management of abiotic stress based on soil management techniques, the use of currently available technologies for irrigation and plant care, the use of materials, nanomaterials, biofertilizers, and growth regulators that can be applied at different stages of plant growth. The application of the mentioned techniques in combination with the use of improved or genetically modified varieties may allow the addition and synergy of different effects in various levels of description of agricultural systems. This synergy is expected to lead to more resilient systems in the face of climate change.

Author details

Hipólito Hernández-Hernández[1], Fabián Pérez-Labrada[1], Ema Laura García Enciso[1], Paola Leija-Martínez[1], Mari Carmen López-Pérez[1], Julia Medrano-Macías[2], Susana González-Morales[3], Antonio Juárez Maldonado[4], Luis Rubén García Dávila[5] and Adalberto Benavides Mendoza[1]*

*Address all correspondence to: abenmen@gmail.com

1 Departamento de Horticultura, Universidad Autónoma Agraria Antonio Narro, Saltillo, México

2 Facultad de Ciencias Biológicas, Universidad Autónoma de Nuevo León, San Nicolás de los Garza, México

3 CONACYT-Universidad Autónoma Agraria Antonio Narro, Saltillo, México

4 Departamento de Botánica, Universidad Autónoma Agraria Antonio Narro, Saltillo, México

5 Cosmocel Brasil, SP, Brasil

References

[1] Adger WN, Dessai S, Goulden M, Hulme M, Lorenzoni I, Nelson DR, Naess LO, Wolf J, Wreford A. Are there social limits to adaptation to climate change? Climatic Change. 2009;**93**:335-354

[2] Olesen JE, Bindi M. Consequences of climate change for European agricultural productivity, land use and policy. European Journal of Agronomy. 2002;**16**:239-262

[3] Clark M, Tilman D. Comparative analysis of environmental impacts of agricultural production systems, agricultural input efficiency, and food choice. Environmental Research Letters. 2017;**12**:64016

[4] Brookes G, Barfoot P. Economic impact of GM crops. GM Crops & Food. 2014;**5**:65-75

[5] Fukushima A, Kusano M, Redestig H, Arita M, Saito K. Integrated omics approaches in plant systems biology. Current Opinion in Chemical Biology. 2009;**13**:532-538

[6] Despommier D. Farming up the city: The rise of urban vertical farms. Trends in Biotechnology. 2013;**31**:388-389

[7] Xu Z, Sun D-W, Zeng X-A, Liu D, Pu H. Research developments in methods to reduce the carbon footprint of the food system: A review. Critical Reviews in Food Science and Nutrition. 2015;**55**:1270-1286

[8] Atkinson NJ, Urwin PE. The interaction of plant biotic and abiotic stresses: From genes to the field. Journal of Experimental Botany. 2012;**63**:3523-3543

[9] Mittler R. Abiotic stress, the field environment and stress combination. Trends in Plant Science. 2006;**11**:15-19

[10] Suzuki N, Rivero RM, Shulaev V, Blumwald E, Mittler R. Abiotic and biotic stress combinations. The New Phytologist. 2014;**203**:32-43

[11] Savvides A, Ali S, Tester M, Fotopoulos V. Chemical priming of plants against multiple abiotic stresses: Mission possible? Trends in Plant Science. 2016;**21**:329-340

[12] Mittler R, Blumwald E. Genetic engineering for modern agriculture: Challenges and perspectives. Annual Review of Plant Biology. 2010;**61**:443-462

[13] Benavides-Mendoza A. Ecophysiology and Biochemistry of Plant Stress. Saltillo, México: Universidad Autónoma Agraria Antonio Narro; 2002

[14] Gates DM. Biophysical Ecology. New York, USA: Springer Verlag; 1980

[15] Awasthi R, Bhandari K, Nayyar H. Temperature stress and redox homeostasis in agricultural crops. Frontiers in Environmental Science. 2015;**3**:11

[16] Liang J, Zhou M, Tobin PC, McGuire AD, Reich PB. Biodiversity influences plant productivity through niche-efficiency. Proceedings of the National Academy of Sciences of the United States of America. 2015;**112**:5738-5743

[17] Gurr GM, Lu Z, Zheng X, Xu H, Zhu P, Chen G, Yao X, Cheng J, Zhu Z, Catindig JL, Villareal S, Van Chien H, Cuong LQ, Channoo C, Chengwattana N, Lan LP, Hai LH, Chaiwong J, Nicol HI, Perovic DJ, Wratten SD, Heong KL. Multi-country evidence that crop diversification promotes ecological intensification of agriculture. Nature Plants. 2016;**2**:16014

[18] Ellis GFR. Top-down causation and emergence: Some comments on mechanisms. Interface Focus. 2011;**2**:1-5

[19] Chapin FS, Bloom AJ, Field CB, Waring RH. Plant responses to multiple environmental factors. Bioscience. 1987;**37**:49-57

[20] Alexieva V, Ivanov S, Sergiev I, Karanov E. Interaction between stresses. Bulgarian Journal of Plant Physiology. 2003;**29**:1-17

[21] Björkman O. High-irradiance stress in higher plants and interaction with other stress factors. In: Biggins J, editor. Progress in Photosynthesis Research. Dordrecht: Springer Netherlands; 1987. pp. 11-18

[22] Terán GE, Benavides A, Hernández F, Quero E. New technologies for horticultural crops. In: Struik PC, Vredenberg WJ, Renkema JA, Parlevliet JE, editors. Plant Production on the Threshold of a New Century. Dordrecht, The Netherlands: Kluwer Academic Publishers; 1994. pp. 375-380

[23] Chapin FS, Matson PA, Vitousek PM. Principles of Terrestrial Ecosystem Ecology. New York, USA: Springer New York; 2011

[24] Krieger-Liszkay A. Singlet oxygen production in photosynthesis. Journal of Experimental Botany. 2004;**56**:337-346

[25] Zhao J, Hartmann H, Trumbore S, Ziegler W, Zhang Y. High temperature causes negative whole-plant carbon balance under mild drought. The New Phytologist. 2013;**200**: 330-339

[26] Pinheiro C, Chaves MM. Photosynthesis and drought: Can we make metabolic connections from available data? Journal of Experimental Botany. 2011;**62**:869-882

[27] Otori K, Tanabe N, Maruyama T, Sato S, Yanagisawa S, Tamoi M, Shigeoka S. Enhanced photosynthetic capacity increases nitrogen metabolism through the coordinated regulation of carbon and nitrogen assimilation in *Arabidopsis thaliana*. Journal of Plant Research. 2017;**130**:909-927

[28] Amtmann A, Armengaud P. Effects of N, P, K and S on metabolism: New knowledge gained from multi-level analysis. Current Opinion in Plant Biology. 2009;**12**:275-283

[29] Kläring H-P, Krumbein A. The effect of constraining the intensity of solar radiation on the photosynthesis, growth, yield and product quality of tomato. Journal of Agronomy and Crop Science. 2013;**199**:351-359

[30] Kuzyakov Y, Gavrichkova O. REVIEW: Time lag between photosynthesis and carbon dioxide efflux from soil: A review of mechanisms and controls. Global Change Biology. 2010;**16**:3386-3406

[31] Schmidt MWI, Torn MS, Abiven S, Dittmar T, Guggenberger G, Janssens IA, Kleber M, Kögel-Knabner I, Lehmann J, Manning DAC, Nannipieri P, Rasse DP, Weiner S, Trumbore SE. Persistence of soil organic matter as an ecosystem property. Nature. 2011; **478**:49-56

[32] Sharif M, Khattak RA, Sarir MS. Effect of different levels of lignitic coal derived humic acid on growth of maize plants. Communications in Soil Science and Plant Analysis. 2002;**33**:3567-3580

[33] Pérez-Labrada F, Benavides-Mendoza A, Valdez-Aguilar LALA, Robledo-Torres V. Citric acid in the nutrient solution increases the mineral absorption in potted tomato grown in calcareous soil. Pakistan Journal of Botany. 2016;**48**:67-74

[34] Niinemets Ü, Sonninen E, Tobias M. Canopy gradients in leaf intercellular CO_2 mole fractions revisited: Interactions between leaf irradiance and water stress need consideration. Plant, Cell and Environment. 2004;**27**:569-583

[35] Diacono M, Montemurro F. Long-term effects of organic amendments on soil fertility. A review. Agronomy for Sustainable Development. 2010;**30**:401-422

[36] Lakshmanan V, Selvaraj G, Bais HP. Functional soil microbiome: Belowground solutions to an aboveground problem. Plant Physiology. 2014;**166**:689-700

[37] Wu X, Ge T, Yuan H, Li B, Zhu H, Zhou P, Sui F, O'Donnell AG, Wu J. Changes in bacterial CO_2 fixation with depth in agricultural soils. Applied Microbiology and Biotechnology. 2014;**98**:2309-2319

[38] Yan D, Wang D, Yang L. Long-term effect of chemical fertilizer, straw, and manure on labile organic matter fractions in a paddy soil. Biology and Fertility of Soils. 2007;**44**: 93-101

[39] Dietz K-J. Efficient high light acclimation involves rapid processes at multiple mechanistic levels. Journal of Experimental Botany. 2015;**66**:2401-2414

[40] Awad J, Stotz HU, Fekete A, Krischke M, Engert C, Havaux M, Berger S, Mueller MJ. 2-cysteine peroxiredoxins and thylakoid ascorbate peroxidase create a water-water cycle that is essential to protect the photosynthetic apparatus under high light stress conditions. Plant Physiology. 2015;**167**:1592-1603

[41] Phee B-K, Cho J-H, Park S, Jung JH, Lee Y-H, Jeon J-S, Bhoo SH, Hahn T-R. Proteomic analysis of the response of Arabidopsis chloroplast proteins to high light stress. Proteomics. 2004;**4**:3560-3568

[42] Hasanuzzaman M, Nahar K, Bhuiyan TF, Anee TI, Inafuku M, Oku H, Fujita M. Salicylic acid: An all-rounder in regulating abiotic stress responses in plants. In: El-Esawi M, editor. Phytohormones - Signaling Mechanisms and Crosstalk in Plant Development and Stress Responses. Rijeka: InTech; 2017

[43] Balal RM, Shahid MA, Javaid MM, Iqbal Z, Anjum MA, Garcia-Sanchez F, Mattson NS. The role of selenium in amelioration of heat-induced oxidative damage in cucumber under high temperature stress. Acta Physiologiae Plantarum. 2016;**38**:158

[44] Maghsoudi K, Emam Y, Pessarakli M. Effect of silicon on photosynthetic gas exchange, photosynthetic pigments, cell membrane stability and relative water content of different wheat cultivars under drought stress conditions. Journal of Plant Nutrition. 2016;**39**: 1001-1015

[45] Zhao H-J, Tan J-F. Role of calcium ion in protection against heat and high irradiance stress-induced oxidative damage to photosynthesis of wheat leaves. Photosynthetica. 2005;**43**:473-476

[46] Morales-Díaz AB, Ortega-Ortíz H, Juárez-Maldonado A, Cadenas-Pliego G, González-Morales S, Benavides-Mendoza A. Application of nanoelements in plant nutrition and its impact in ecosystems. Advances in Natural Sciences: Nanoscience and Nanotechnology. 2017;**8**:13001

[47] Cantore V, Pace B, Albrizio R. Kaolin-based particle film technology affects tomato physiology, yield and quality. Environmental and Experimental Botany. 2009;**66**:279-288

[48] Erez A, Glenn DM. The effect of particle film technology on yield and fruit quality. Acta Horticulturae. 2004;**636**:505-508

[49] Maiti RK, de la Rosa-Ibarra M, Sandoval ND. Genotypic variability in glossy Sorghum lines for resistance to drought, salinity and temperature stress at the seedling stage. Journal of Plant Physiology. 1994;**143**:241-244

[50] Lee SS, Shah HS, Awad YM, Kumar S, Ok YS. Synergy effects of biochar and polyacrylamide on plants growth and soil erosion control. Environment and Earth Science. 2015;**74**:2463-2473

[51] Lenton TM, Crouch M, Johnson M, Pires N, Dolan L. First plants cooled the Ordovician. Nature Geoscience. 2012;**5**:86-89

[52] Wagner D, Przybyla D, op den Camp R, Kim C, Landgraf F, Lee KP, Würsch M, Laloi C, Nater M, Hideg E, Apel K. The genetic basis of singlet oxygen–induced stress responses of *Arabidopsis thaliana*. Science (80-.). 2004;**306**:1183-1185

[53] Teixeira EI, Fischer G, Van Velthuizen H, Walter C, Ewert F. Global hot-spots of heat stress on agricultural crops due to climate change. Agricultural and Forest Meteorology. 2013;**170**:206-215

[54] Prasad PVV, Boote KJ, Allen LH. Adverse high temperature effects on pollen viability, seed-set, seed yield and harvest index of grain-sorghum [*Sorghum bicolor* (L.) Moench] are more severe at elevated carbon dioxide due to higher tissue temperatures. Agricultural and Forest Meteorology. 2006;**139**:237-251

[55] Carvalho LC, Coito JL, Colaço S, Sangiogo M, Amâncio S. Heat stress in grapevine: The pros and cons of acclimation. Plant, Cell and Environment. 2015;**38**:777-789

[56] Bita CE, Gerats T. Plant tolerance to high temperature in a changing environment: Scientific fundamentals and production of heat stress-tolerant crops. Frontiers in Plant Science. 2013;**4**:1-18

[57] Hasanuzzaman M, Nahar K, Alam MM, Roychowdhury R, Fujita M. Physiological, biochemical, and molecular mechanisms of heat stress tolerance in plants. International Journal of Molecular Sciences. 2013;**14**:9643-9684

[58] Yabuta Y. Functions of heat shock transcription factors involved in response to photo-oxidative stresses in Arabidopsis. Bioscience, Biotechnology, and Biochemistry. 2016; **8451**:1-10

[59] Wani SH, Kumar V, Shriram V, Sah SK. Phytohormones and their metabolic engineering for abiotic stress tolerance in crop plants. The Crop Journal. 2016;**4**:162-176

[60] Jagadish SVK, Muthurajan R, Oane R, Wheeler TR, Heuer S, Bennett J, Craufurd PQ. Physiological and proteomic approaches to address heat tolerance during anthesis in rice (*Oryza sativa* L.). Journal of Experimental Botany. 2010;**61**:143-156

[61] Qi M, Liu Y, Li T. Nano-TiO_2 improve the photosynthesis of tomato leaves under mild heat stress. Biological Trace Element Research. 2013;**156**:323-328

[62] Zhao L, Peng B, Hernandez-Viezcas JA, Rico C, Sun Y, Peralta-Videa JR. Stress response and tolerance of *Zea mays* to CeO_2 nanoparticles: Cross talk among H_2O_2, heat shock protein, and lipid peroxidation. ACS Nano. 2012;**2012**:9615